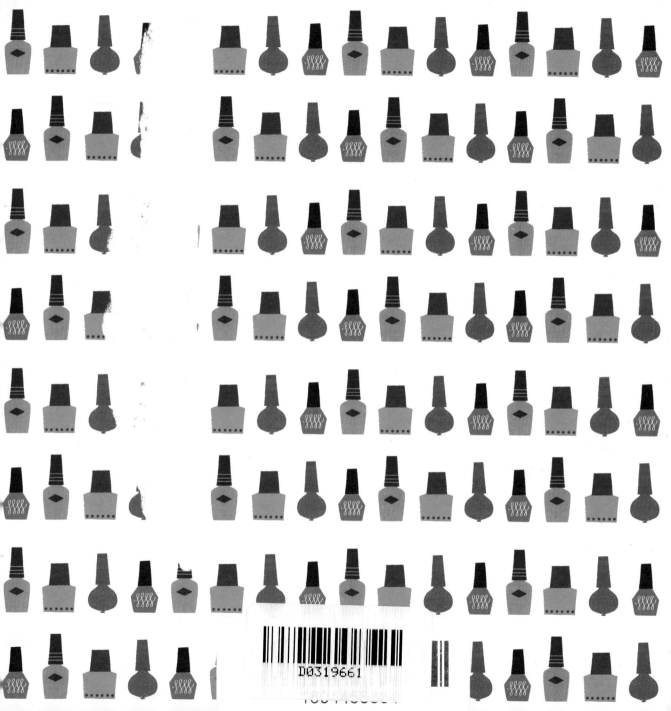

Nail Candy

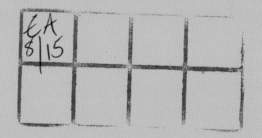

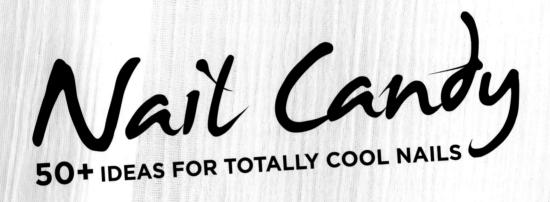

Nail Candy

50+ IDEAS FOR TOTALLY COOL NAILS

NAIL ART & TEXT
DONNE & GINNY GEER

PHOTOGRAPHS
NICOLE HILL GERULAT

PROP STYLING
MALLORY ULLMAN

ILLUSTRATIONS
DEBBIE POWELL

weldon**owen**

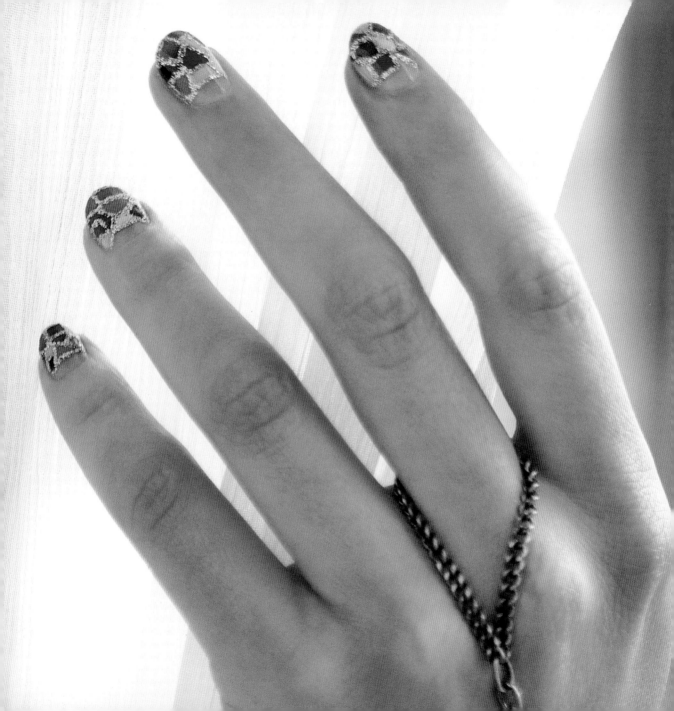

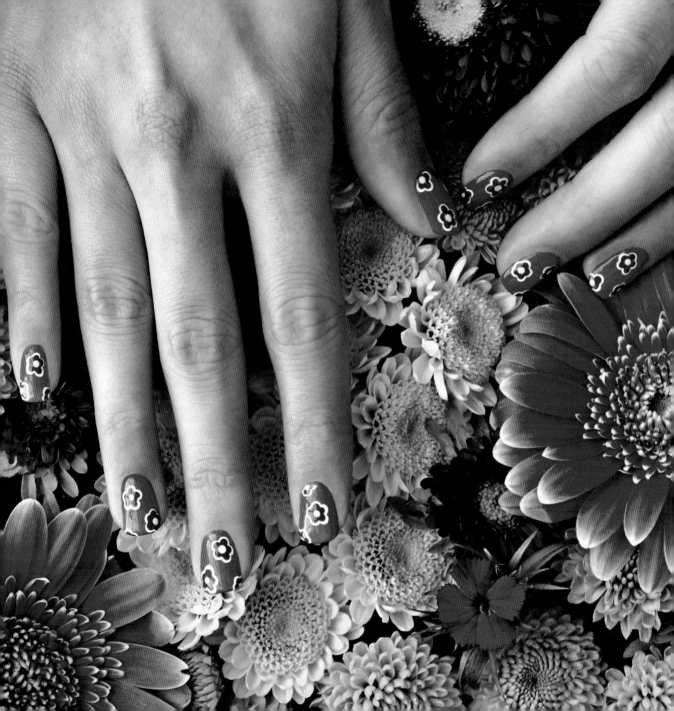

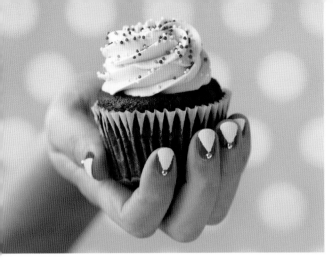
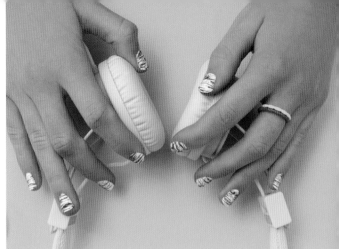

NAILCARE BASICS

MANI MANIA

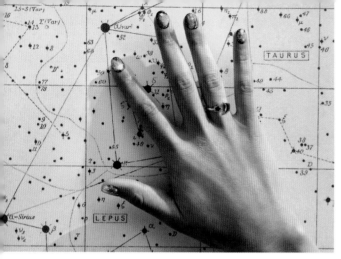
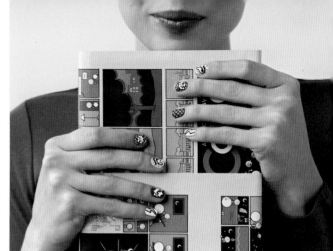

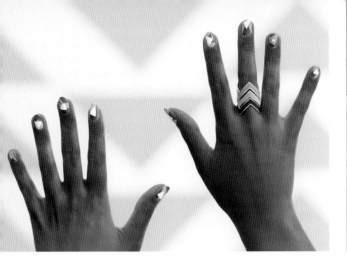
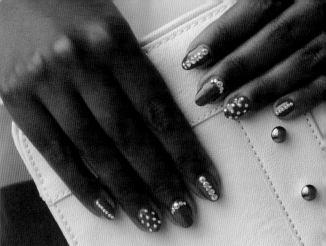

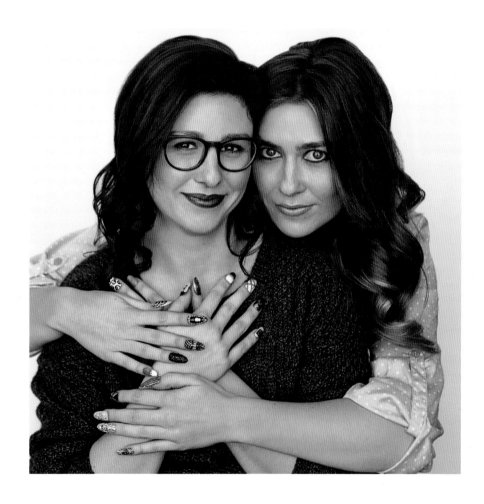

This book is dedicated to our mother. Thank you for giving us life, love, and fingernails!

A Note

FROM THE AUTHORS

As sisters, our relationship has always had its ups and downs, but the one thing that never fails to pull us together is our love of nail art. Growing up, we looked to our mother for nail inspiration—sure, we may have found her collection of red and pink polish a little boring, and she often rolled her eyes at the outrageous colors we liked best. But Mom always showed her support for our habit by lending us her coveted fast-drying topcoat. Fast-forward 20 years, and she still shows her support—not just for us as her daughters, but also for our work as creative directors of Hey, Nice Nails, our very own nail salon in Long Beach.

Trust us, we didn't start out as the nail artists we are now! We got here through clouds of acetone vapors and flooded cuticles. Blogging gave us an outlet to share our favorite manicures, play around with new techniques, and gather inspiration from the recent explosion of nail-art ideas. From the blog came an online shop, a gig painting manis at a local speakeasy (everyone starts somewhere!), and involvement in a growing community of nail-art nuts. Then one day we made our love affair with nails official: We got licensed as beauty professionals, opened up shop, and brought our manis to the masses.

Painting art on your fingertips turns a part of your body into a statement-making accessory, and each of the projects in this book is a chance to transform your nails into ten tiny canvases. From easy designs that you can doodle on during commercial breaks to more ambitious hand-painted looks that'll take some time, there's something for everyone in these pages! We give you permission to take these techniques and make them your own—to experiment, make a mess, and develop your own signature nail styles, just like we did.

Nail Candy represents a totally disposable art form and a playful means of self-expression that lifts your spirits and won't break the bank. The joy of a fresh, well-painted manicure is a small luxury that all women can appreciate, especially when someone stops you and says, "Hey, nice nails!"

XOXO
Gin & Donne ♡

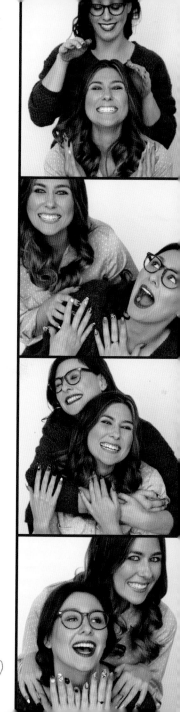

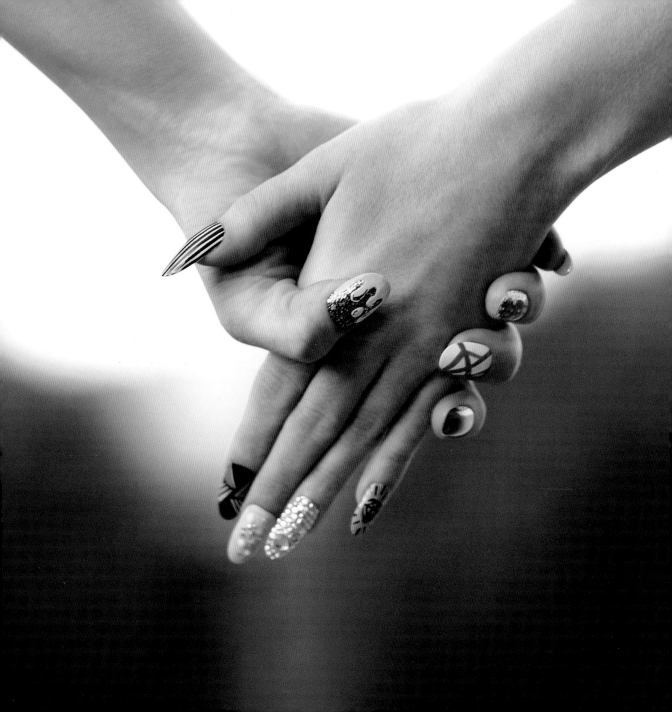

*We hope this book inspires you
to make the most of your manis,
whether you're a nail-art noob or
a seasoned lacquer veteran!*

Nailcare Basics

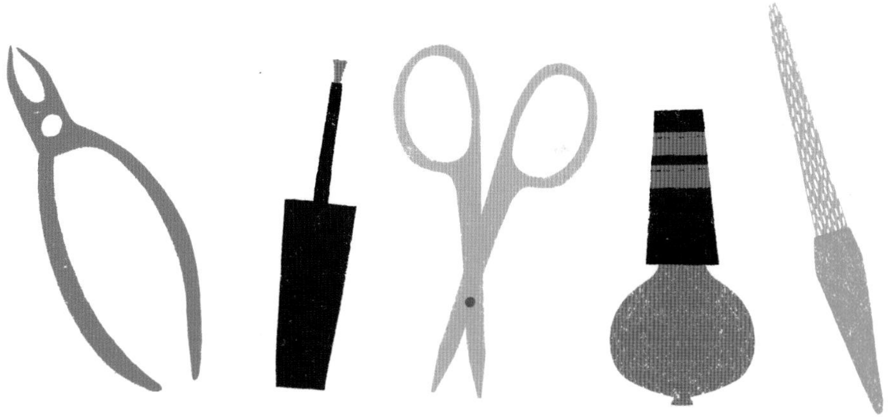

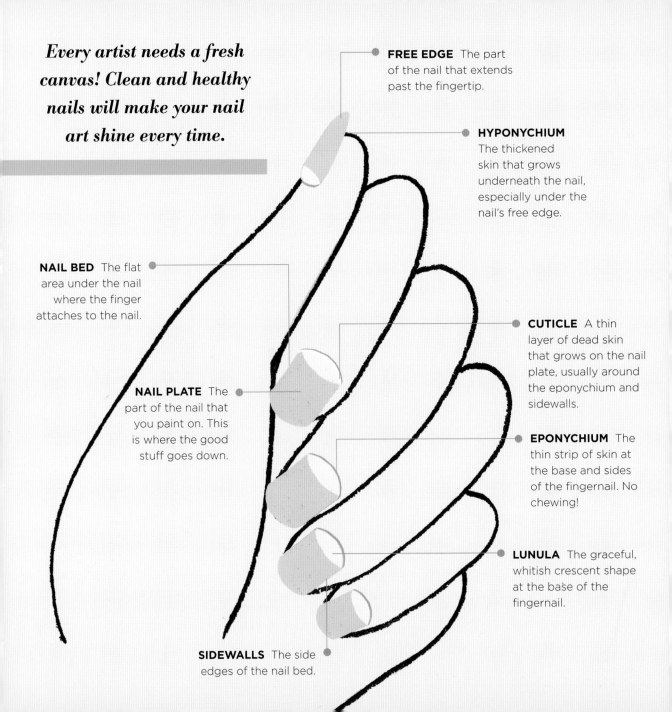

Every artist needs a fresh canvas! Clean and healthy nails will make your nail art shine every time.

FREE EDGE The part of the nail that extends past the fingertip.

HYPONYCHIUM The thickened skin that grows underneath the nail, especially under the nail's free edge.

NAIL BED The flat area under the nail where the finger attaches to the nail.

CUTICLE A thin layer of dead skin that grows on the nail plate, usually around the eponychium and sidewalls.

NAIL PLATE The part of the nail that you paint on. This is where the good stuff goes down.

EPONYCHIUM The thin strip of skin at the base and sides of the fingernail. No chewing!

LUNULA The graceful, whitish crescent shape at the base of the fingernail.

SIDEWALLS The side edges of the nail bed.

PREP YOUR NAILS FOR A

Perfect Mani'

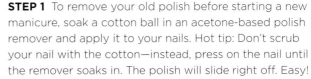

MATERIALS

COTTON BALLS

POLISH REMOVER

ANTIBACTERIAL SOAP

NAIL BRUSH

ORANGEWOOD OR PLASTIC
CUTICLE PUSHER

CHEMICAL CUTICLE REMOVER

CUTICLE NIPPERS

CUTICLE OIL

MOISTURIZER

ACETONE

STEP 1 To remove your old polish before starting a new manicure, soak a cotton ball in an acetone-based polish remover and apply it to your nails. Hot tip: Don't scrub your nail with the cotton—instead, press on the nail until the remover soaks in. The polish will slide right off. Easy!

STEP 2 Wash your hands with a mild antibacterial soap and warm water. Use a brush to scrub underneath the nails and along the sides to remove any traces of oil or dirt.

STEP 3 Be sweet to your cuticles: Gently use an orangewood or a plastic cuticle pusher to push back any skin growing on the nail plate. If you have stubborn or overgrown cuticles, apply a chemical cuticle remover according to the manufacturer's directions.

STEP 4 If you have any hangnails or pieces of skin that are loose or jagged, snip them off carefully using your cuticle nippers. Be very careful not to pull on the skin as you trim or you'll hurt yourself—cuticles are delicate business.

STEP 5 Wash your hands again with soap and warm water, then apply cuticle oil to the areas where you pushed or nipped for an intense boost of hydration. Be sure to moisturize your hands with your favorite lotion, too. Dry cuticles are the enemy of excellent nail art!

STEP 6 Before you paint, use a cotton ball soaked in acetone to clean the nails—this prevents the polish from chipping or peeling, making your mani go the extra mile.

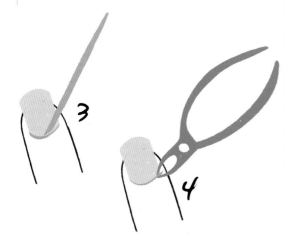

CUTICLE OIL Nourishes cuticles after you tame them with a cuticle pusher.

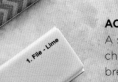

ACETONE A strong chemical that breaks down nail polish. Moisturize after use!

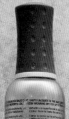

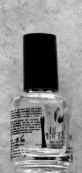

TOPCOAT

BASECOAT

EMERY BOARD & BUFFER

COTTON BALLS

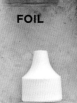

FOIL

GLITTER

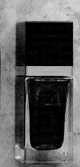

SHIMMER

NAIL CLIPPERS

POLISH REMOVER A dissolvent that breaks down nail polish. Don't inhale!

CUTICLE NIPPERS Trims hanging or jagged skin around the nail.

CUTICLE REMOVER A chemical that removes tough skin from the cuticle area.

ORANGEWOOD CUTICLE PUSHER Pushes back soft skin growing on the nail plate.

NAIL BRUSH

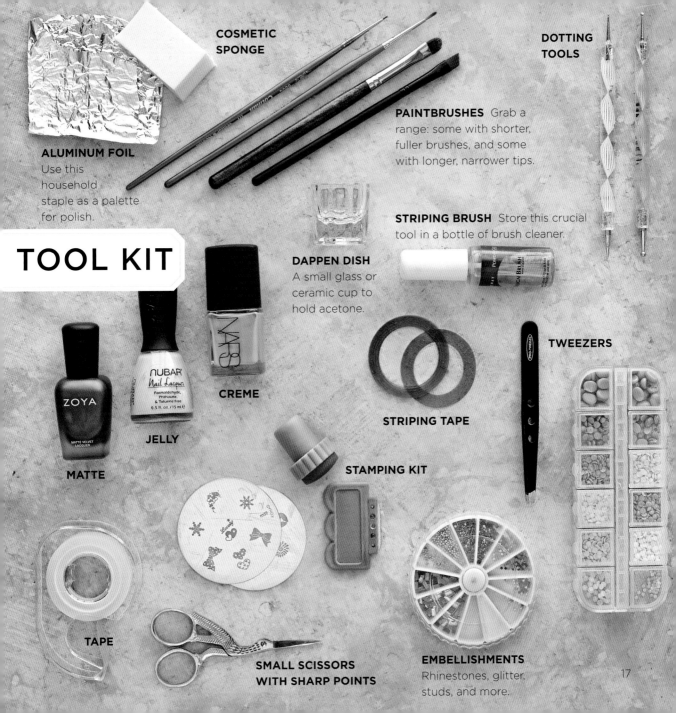

COSMETIC SPONGE

DOTTING TOOLS

PAINTBRUSHES Grab a range: some with shorter, fuller brushes, and some with longer, narrower tips.

ALUMINUM FOIL Use this household staple as a palette for polish.

TOOL KIT

DAPPEN DISH A small glass or ceramic cup to hold acetone.

STRIPING BRUSH Store this crucial tool in a bottle of brush cleaner.

CREME

JELLY

MATTE

STRIPING TAPE

TWEEZERS

STAMPING KIT

TAPE

SMALL SCISSORS WITH SHARP POINTS

EMBELLISHMENTS Rhinestones, glitter, studs, and more.

17

Find the shape that suits your hand, your mani, and your mood.

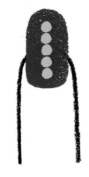

ROUND

For a natural look on short nails, opt for a rounded tip. This reliable shape is easy to maintain, and one size fits all.

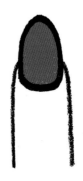

OVAL

Gently tapering in from the sidewalls is flattering and elongating on almost everyone. Think of these shapes as high heels for your nails.

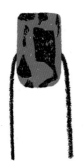

SQUARE

A blunt free edge and straight sidewalls make a striking shape on long fingers. For a perfect square, hold the file flat and perpendicular to your fingertip.

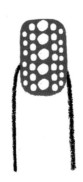

SQUOVAL

Combine the elegance of an oval nail with the durability of a square shape. Like the round shape, this effect flatters any finger.

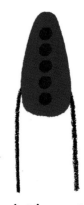

POINTED

This dramatic, tapered nail shape instantly lengthens each finger. It might not be a Tuesday-at-the-office look, but it sure can take an avant-garde mani to the next level.

Shape & File

FOR FABULOUS FINGERNAILS

MATERIALS

NAIL CLIPPERS

FINE- OR MEDIUM-GRIT NAIL FILE

BUFFER

STEP 1 Before you even consider picking up a nail file, make sure your nails are completely dry—wet nails will tear or break if filed.

STEP 2 If you're taking length off your nails, gently trim the nails with clippers first to save yourself some time.

STEP 3 Decide on a shape. If you're not sure where to start, use the shape of your cuticle as a guide for the free edge of your nails to create pretty symmetry—or look to your left for a host of shape choices!

STEP 4 For each nail, hold the nail file at a 45-degree angle and slightly stroke the file from the corner to the center repeatedly in one direction. Then switch directions to file from the other corner back to the center. Never use a back-and-forth sawing motion—you risk creating uneven shapes or damaging your nail.

STEP 5 Grab a buffer and rub the top of your nail bed and the edges of your nails. This will level off any ridges in your nail, creating a smooth surface for painting and adding a natural shine.

Polish Perfectly

EVERY TIME

STEP 1 By the end of this book you'll have read this countless times, but that's because we mean it! Start every mani (whether a fancy design or just a pretty polish) by applying basecoat over clean nails. We call this doing your ABCs: Applying basecoat.

STEP 2 Open up your basecoat and wipe the bottle brush on the insides of the bottle's neck to remove excess polish, which will flood your cuticles and make everything messy. Avoid wiping polish on the top of the bottle; this will keep your bottles tidy.

STEP 3 Now it's time to use that basecoat. We always paint our dominant hand first, as it keeps us motivated. Hold your brush over your first nail and let a bead of polish form at the brush's tip. You should have just enough polish to cover the nail completely.

STEP 4 Working quickly and lightly, drop the bead of polish in the nail's center. Push the polish down the nail toward the cuticle.

STEP 5 Press down lightly on the brush to fan its bristles, making an even line at the base of the nail.

STEP 6 Sweep the brush toward one sidewall, then put some pressure on the brush and pull it straight up and off the nail tip in one continuous motion.

STEP 7 Return to the cuticle and draw the brush along the other sidewall and up toward the tip. If polish floods your cuticles or

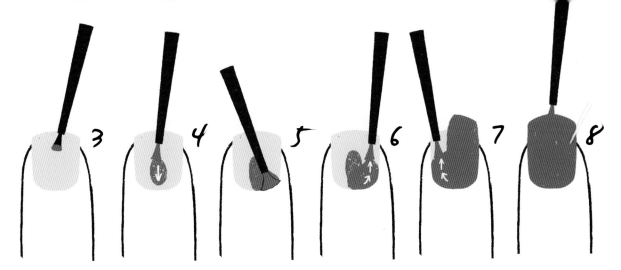

sidewalls, stop and wipe your brush. You can also point your fingers downward, making the polish stream toward the tips.

STEP 8 Go back and gently press the brush in the nail's center, then lightly and quickly brush over the entire nail to distribute the basecoat in a nice, even layer. Now that you've finished one nail, go ahead and hit up your others. Let them dry.

STEP 9 Congratulations, your clear basecoat is complete! Now go ahead and add your colored polish using the exact same painting technique.

STEP 10 Once your colored polish dries, your nails are ready for clear topcoat—so don't ever forget it! Clear topcoat locks in color and minimizes the appearance of brushstrokes. For nail art that lasts, add a fresh layer every few days.

STEP 11 If you've got bloopers, fill a dappen dish with acetone, dip the angled brush in it, and erase any mini messes on your nails.

STEP 12 Moisturize your hands with your fave cuticle oil and lotion and survey your style. See? You nailed it.

For extra steadiness, tuck your painting arm in close to your waist, and rest its hand or pinky finger on a stable surface.

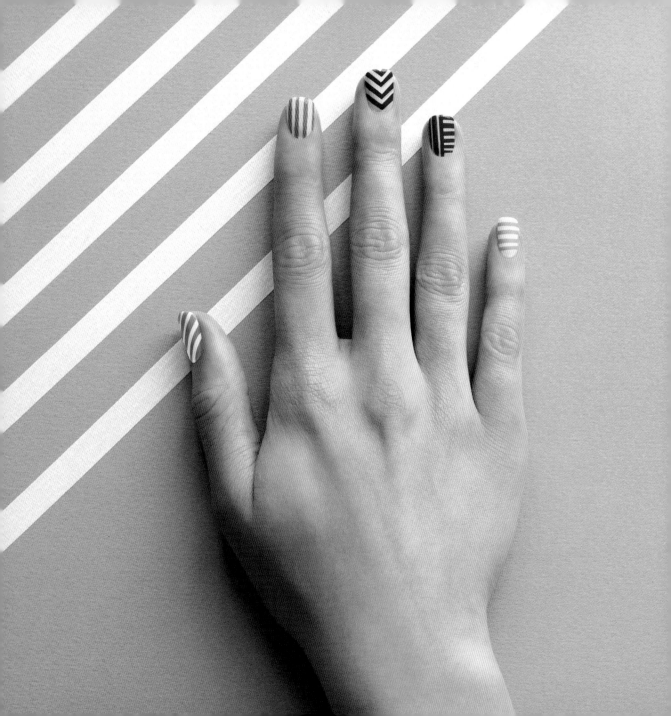

MASTER
Color & Pattern
COMBOS

SKIN-TONE SAVVY

So your basecoat is dry and ready for nail art. Which base color should you go for? Consider your skin tone—the same way you would for a dress or lipstick—for nail art that flatters. Chilly colors like blues and purples will flatter skin with cool undertones, while orange and red colors are warm hues that will complement a warm complexion.

COLOR-THEORY BASICS

Think back on the color wheel from elementary school when planning a multi-hued manicure—it'll help you pick combinations that look amazing together. Pairing analogous shades (colors that are next to each other on the color wheel, like purple and blue) will create a harmonious look. Complementary colors (those that are directly across from each other on the color wheel, like yellow and purple) yield eye-catching contrast.

PICKING A DESIGN VIBE

Pick a motif that says what you're all about. Straight, clean lines have a bold and fresh look, while curves, swoops, and blends feel more feminine and soft. Generally, stick with bold or soft designs in any given mani—that way you can mix up the design from nail to nail without making it feel schizophrenic.

IT'S ALL IN THE MIX

There's a science to pairing color schemes and patterns. A wild pattern can feel more cohesive when executed with tried-and-true combos, like analogous or complementary colors. Or go the opposite route: Mix it up with a rainbow of random color combos, but use a consistent pattern to harmonize your look.

MINDING THE GAPS

It's not just what you paint, it's also where you paint—and where you don't. Your mani will look best if there's approximately the same amount of negative space on each nail. For example: Go nuts switching up the directionality of lines and placement of shapes, but leave about the same amount of space between each of the lines and shapes in your pattern. Controlled chaos!

TRY YOUR HAND AT IT

Now go for it—dots, zigzags, swirls, straight lines, and geometric shapes are yours to explore. As long as you're having fun, you can't go wrong.

Pause before you polish to think about color and pattern—it'll really amp up your nail art's impact.

DESIGN YOUR OWN *Custom Sets*

MATERIALS

- SET OF FULL-COVERAGE NAIL TIPS
- NAIL FILE & BUFFER
- ORANGEWOOD STICK
- DOUBLE-SIDED TAPE
- CLEAR BASECOAT
- POLISH
- WHATEVER ELSE YOU'RE USING TO DECORATE
- CLEAR TOPCOAT
- NAIL GLUE

To paint tricky patterns, save time, or create a reusable mani, go with an acrylic set. Fake it 'til you make it, ladies!

STEP 1 It's all in the fit! Find nail tips that are about the same size and shape as your pinkies, then try a size up on each nail closer to your thumb. If you find you're in between sizes, just file the tips until they're a perfect fit.

STEP 2 Use a file and buffer to work the tips into your desired shape and smooth out any bumps or rough edges.

STEP 3 Affix your nail tips to an orangewood stick or pencil using double-sided tape. This will hold them steady while you decorate them to your heart's content. Just think: You won't have to paint with your nondominant hand!

STEP 4 Paint each plastic tip as you would your own fingernail, starting with a clear basecoat and then a layer of the polish of your choice. Let that dry and add any fanciness you've got in mind—embellishments or tricky hand-painted designs. Apply a quick-dry topcoat to your set once they're done.

STEP 5 To put on your tips, work with just one at a time. Begin with the pinky nail of your dominant hand and place a small drop of glue toward the base of the first nail, making sure not to flood the cuticle. Carefully position and then press the artificial nail onto your nail bed. Hold and apply moderate pressure for 30 seconds.

STEP 6 Working from pinkies to thumbs, repeat these steps until each hand is dressed up in fashionable fakes.

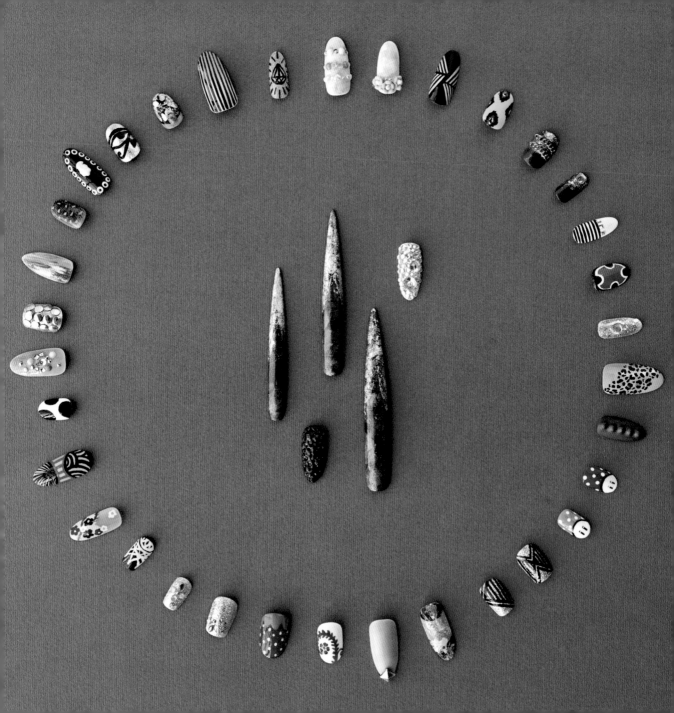

Manì Manìa

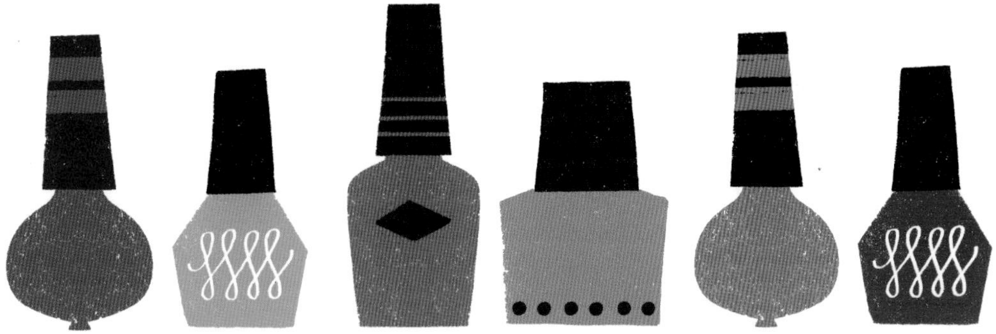

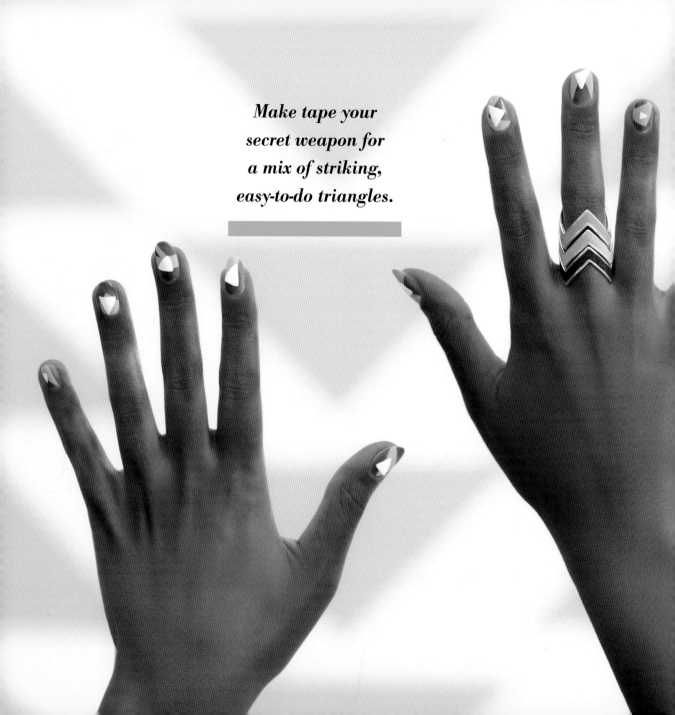

Make tape your secret weapon for a mix of striking, easy-to-do triangles.

SHAPE TAPE FOR A
Geometry Lesson

STEP 1 Start with your ABCs: Apply basecoat and let it dry. Then lay on a base color—we chose a bubbly seafoam green.

STEP 2 With dry nails, rip off lots of tiny tape pieces. Use scissors to trim the pieces' raw edges so you get a nice clean line when you stick the tape on your nails. No special tape necessary: We used the regular old sticky stuff.

STEP 3 Press each piece of tape on the palm of your hand to dial down the stickiness, then tape off areas of your nails where you want the base color to show through. Vary the shapes on each nail—it's fun to create different sizes of triangles, or even a rectangle or two. Hot tip: Press firmly on the edges of the tape so no polish seeps underneath.

STEP 4 Pick a color to contrast with your first (like this sassy cerulean). Coat your nails, tape and all.

STEP 5 Remove the tape immediately but gently. Once your nails are dry (no cheating), you're ready for another round of tape, if you've got the patience. Tape over the places where you want to see your first two colors of polish peeking through, and paint each nail with your third color. White pops against these ocean tones—in fact, white pops with anything!

STEP 6 Peel off the tape again, and (once it's dry) seal in your electric masterpiece with a clear topcoat.

MATERIALS

BASECOAT

SEAFOAM GREEN, CERULEAN & WHITE POLISH

TAPE

SCISSORS

CLEAR TOPCOAT

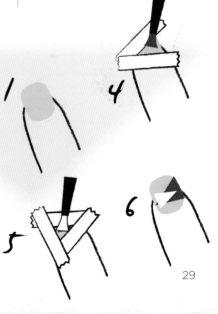

29

FADE INTO *Ombre*

STEP 1 Basecoat it up, then douse your nails in the color you want to show at the cuticle, like this icy turquoise.

STEP 2 Pour a strip of this color onto some foil and quickly add a strip of your contrasting color (like this dreamy lilac) next to it. Use a toothpick to blend the two polishes together just at the edges where they meet.

STEP 3 Press the flat side of your cosmetic sponge firmly into the polish on the foil, blending the polishes together more and soaking up the mix. The sponge will function almost like a stamp, transferring the blended color from the foil to your fingernail.

STEP 4 After your nails have dried, dab the sponge onto the first nail with the turquoise at your cuticle and the lilac at your tip. Sponge-paint all your nails, adding polish to the foil as needed to keep the polish wet so you can work with it.

STEP 5 If your color gradient is not as dramatic as you would like, persist and sponge again! It may take a few coats for the effect to become as bold as you are.

STEP 6 With dry 'tips, clean areas around the skin and cuticle with an angled brush dipped in acetone.

STEP 7 After your polish dries, seal in your design with a layer of every mani's BFF—a glossy clear topcoat.

MATERIALS

BASECOAT

TURQUOISE & LILAC POLISH

ALUMINUM FOIL

TOOTHPICK

COSMETIC SPONGE

ANGLED BRUSH

DAPPEN DISH

ACETONE

CLEAR TOPCOAT

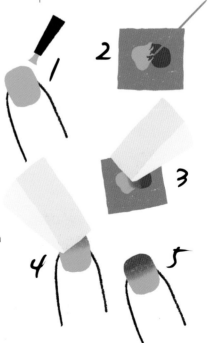

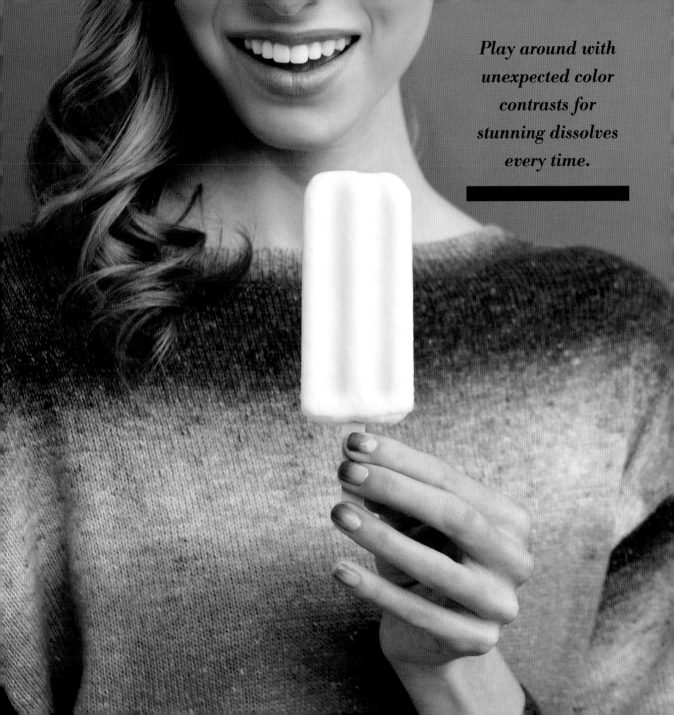

Play around with unexpected color contrasts for stunning dissolves every time.

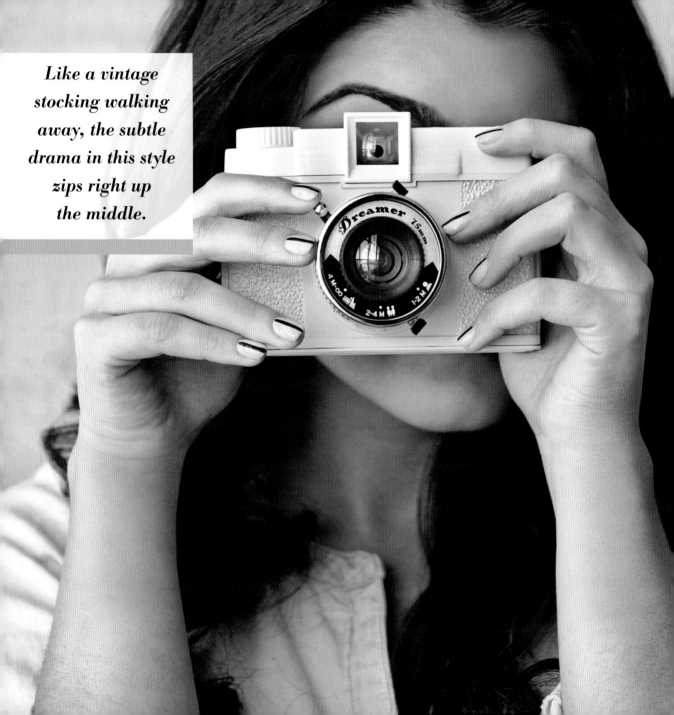

Like a vintage stocking walking away, the subtle drama in this style zips right up the middle.

SLASH ON SOME

Sassy Seams

MATERIALS

BASECOAT

NUDE & BLACK POLISH

STRIPING BRUSH

CLEAR TOPCOAT

STEP 1 ABC (apply basecoat). After it's dry, slick a nude color onto your 'tips and let it dry, too. Hot tip: Match your polish to your skin tone to make this mani extra subtle and classy and to give the illusion of longer fingers.

STEP 2 Dip your striping brush into your bottle of black polish, wiping excess polish off on the bottle's neck. Note that the more polish on the brush, the thicker your stripes will be.

STEP 3 Place the tip of the striping brush close to the cuticle of your first nail. With gentle, even pressure, lay the brush flat onto the nail and pull it straight out and off the tip. Stripe the rest of your nails.

STEP 4 When your stripes are dry, slick on a clear topcoat. This is one quietly arresting look that's ready for its close-up!

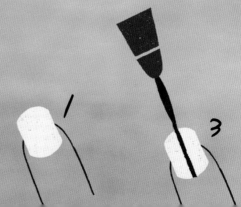

BELIEVE THE
Stripe Hype

STEP 1 Start with a dry basecoat. Then select the lightest color of polish from your chosen palette (like our pale pink or yellow) and use it as a base color on all your nails. Let it dry.

STEP 2 Dip your striping brush in your next polish. Tap the striping brush's tip on the inside of the bottle to remove excess polish—this will allow you maximum control over the size of your stripes.

STEP 3 Start your first zigzag by placing the striping brush in the middle of a nail. Pressing evenly along the nail, pull the brush straight out and off the tip.

STEP 4 To finish the zigzag, place the striping brush at the middle of the nail again, but this time rotate it horizontally across the nail. Lay it flat and pull it straight toward the nail wall and off the nail. Use this color to make a stripe on each of your nails.

STEP 5 When your first zigzags are dry, rinse your brush and add a new color next to the first color using the same brush motion and even pressure. Keep the colors contrasting so that they pop—this mix of pale pink, yellow, and light blue makes the black, dark blue, red, and purple really shout.

STEP 6 Repeat until your nails are fully, fabulously striped and dry, and seal the deal with a clear topcoat.

MATERIALS

BASECOAT

PALE PINK, RED, BLACK, DARK BLUE, LIGHT BLUE, YELLOW & PURPLE POLISH

STRIPING BRUSH

CLEAR TOPCOAT

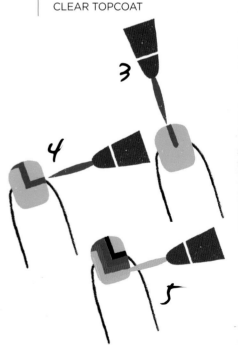

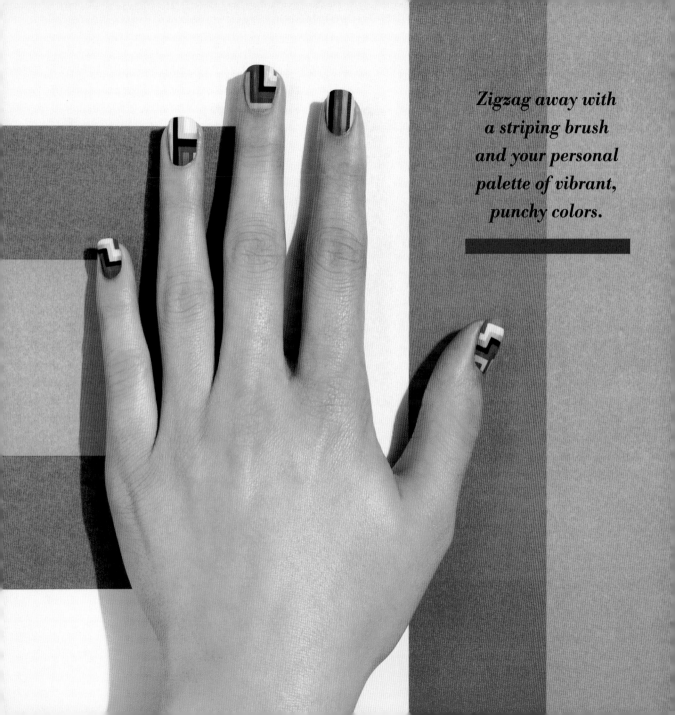

Zigzag away with a striping brush and your personal palette of vibrant, punchy colors.

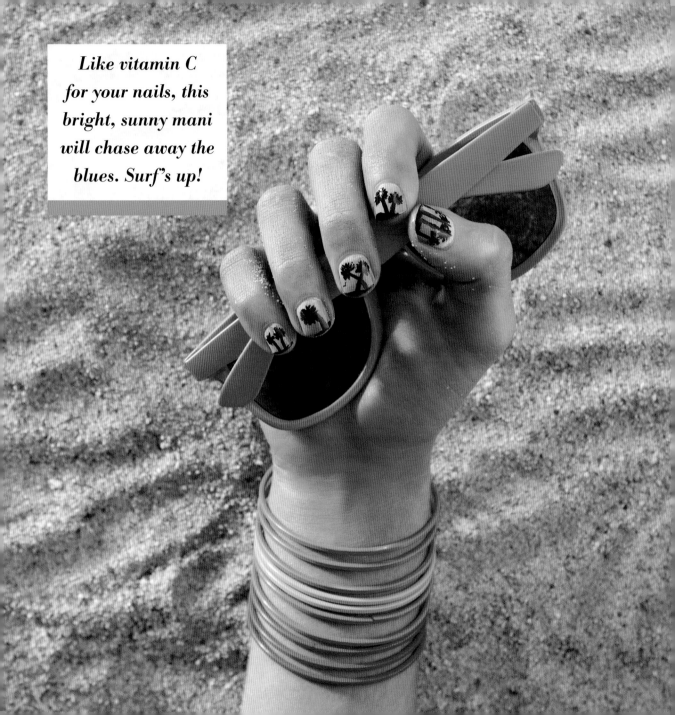

Like vitamin C for your nails, this bright, sunny mani will chase away the blues. Surf's up!

DAYDREAM ON THE BEACH IN *Sunset* SILHOUETTES

MATERIALS

- BASECOAT
- YELLOW, ORANGE, PINK, PURPLE & BLACK POLISH
- ALUMINUM FOIL
- TOOTHPICK
- COSMETIC SPONGE
- SMALL, ROUND PAINTBRUSH
- ANGLED BRUSH
- ACETONE
- DAPPEN DISH
- CLEAR TOPCOAT

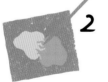

STEP 1 As usual, ABC (apply basecoat) and let it dry. Give your nails a warm yellow wash—this will be the backdrop for your ombre sunset.

STEP 2 After your yellow coat dries, dump a puddle of yellow polish on a piece of aluminum foil and add a puddle of orange polish next to it. At the edge where the colors meet, blend them with a toothpick.

STEP 3 Dab a cosmetic sponge into the paint to pick up the gradient, and sponge it onto the base of your nails.

STEP 4 When your nails are dry, repeat with pink and purple polish. Sponge the pink-to-purple gradient onto your nails toward the free edge, overlapping slightly with the orange polish in the center of the nail. Let your sunsets dry, then use an angled brush dipped in acetone to tidy up any stray polish on your skin.

STEP 5 Puddle black polish onto the foil and dip in the small, round paintbrush. Swipe the paintbrush across each nail's free edge to create a beach. Then paint the palm trees' trunks onto each nail, making the trunks sway and cross for an especially nice view. You can also mix up the number of trees on each nail.

STEP 6 Then, with quick, light strokes, radiate tiny lines in a circle to create leafy tops. Finally, use your small brush to complete the scene with a tiny seagull, like you see on the middle finger in our photo. Let your nails dry, add your clear topcoat, and throw on your shades.

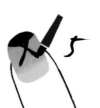

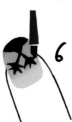

SOAK UP PATTERN WITH A
Simple Stamp

MATERIALS

BASECOAT

YELLOW, LIME GREEN, ORANGE & PINK POLISH

NAIL STAMPING KIT (PLATE, SCRAPER & RUBBER STAMP)

ACETONE

LINT-FREE PAD

PAPER TOWELS

CLEAR TOPCOAT

STEP 1 Start with a basic manicure in a snappy yellow over a dry basecoat. Then grab a nail stamping kit, which comes with a rubber stamp, scraper, and stamping plates engraved with ready-made designs. To prep your tools, pick a stamping plate and wipe it down with acetone and a lint-free pad.

STEP 2 Once you're dry, lay down a few paper towels under your stamping plates. Brush some contrasting polish (like this fresh lime green) on the plate over the design.

STEP 3 To remove excess polish, hold the scraper at a 45-degree angle and firmly scrape the polish across the engraved design and off the plate. Hot tip: Too much polish covering your design will turn your nails into a hot mess.

STEP 4 Using the stamp, pick up the design by slowly rolling the rubber top over the polish-covered area on the plate.

STEP 5 Stamp the design onto each nail with the same rolling technique. Repeat with as many hues as your nails can handle, rinsing the stamp and letting your nails dry between colors.

STEP 6 Finish your dry mani with clear topcoat.

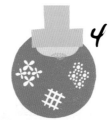

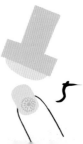

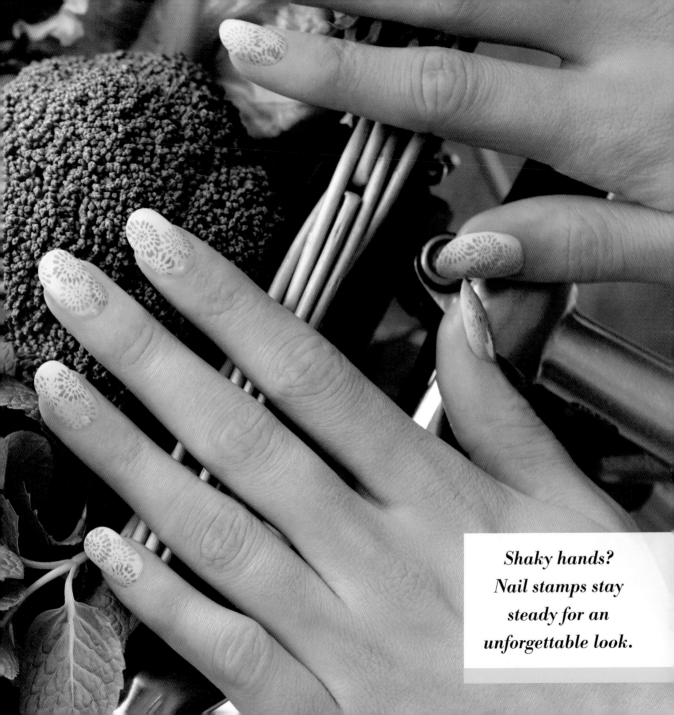

Shaky hands?
Nail stamps stay
steady for an
unforgettable look.

SPARKLE & STUN IN A
Studded STYLE

STEP 1 Start with a basecoat. When it's dry, layer on a base color in a deep magenta hue.

STEP 2 Lay out your studs on a flat surface, and start designing the layout for each nail using studs of slightly different sizes. You could vary vertical and horizontal lines of studs, cover the nail completely, or even just outline the cuticle or free edge.

STEP 3 When your nails are dry, place some clear topcoat on a piece of aluminum foil. With your dotting tool, dab a drop of topcoat onto a nail where you want to place a stud.

STEP 4 With the dotting tool, pick up a stud from one of your designs and press it into the drop of topcoat.

STEP 5 Repeat on all your nails until you're digging the stud pattern. After your nails dry, slowly and gently paint clear topcoat over each nail and its studs to lock in your naughty-but-nice look. Bling-a-ding-ding!

MATERIALS

- BASECOAT
- MAGENTA POLISH
- ROUND STUDS IN VARIOUS SIZES
- CLEAR TOPCOAT
- ALUMINUM FOIL
- DOTTING TOOL

Bedazzle your nails in a pattern that mixes pretty and tough as well as you do.

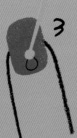 3

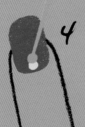 4

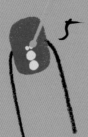 5

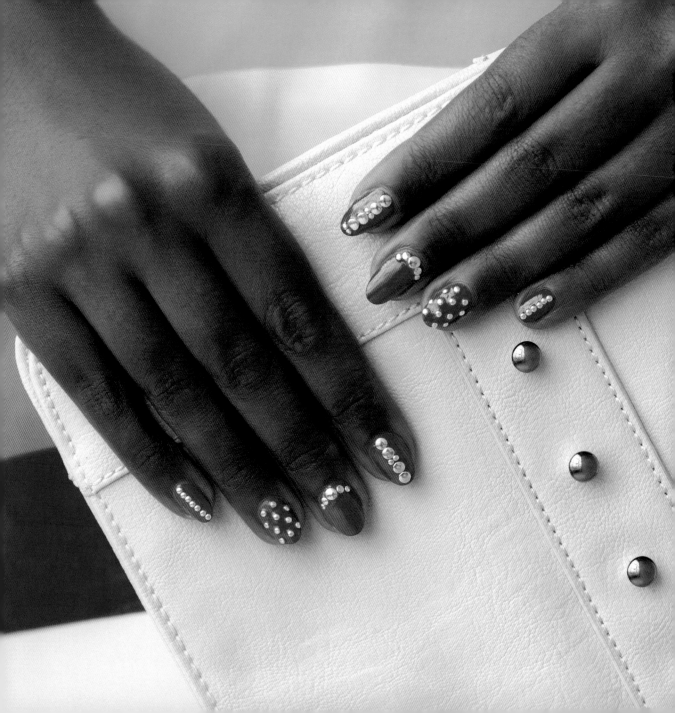

PURR OUT LOUD IN

Leopard Prints

MATERIALS

BASECOAT

CHERRY RED, WHITE & BLACK POLISH

ALUMINUM FOIL

SMALL, ROUND PAINTBRUSH

CLEAR TOPCOAT

Take your nails for a walk on the wild side with a schizophrenic style that roars.

STEP 1 Start by painting your nails cherry red over a dry basecoat. When that's dry, cover half of each red nail with white.

STEP 2 Dribble a little red polish onto a piece of aluminum foil and pick some up with your small, round paintbrush.

STEP 3 Gently dab the red-dipped paintbrush in the white area of your first nail to create tiny dots—these are the centers of your soon-to-be leopard spots. Dab these rosettes on all your nails.

STEP 4 After your nails dry, rinse your paintbrush and add black polish to your foil palette. Dip the brush into the black polish, then slowly press the brush's top edge along the side of a red dot. Just barely lift the brush off the nail, allowing some polish to drizzle along the dot's perimeter. Continue dabbing and drizzling to make tiny, imperfect half-circles around the red dots.

STEP 5 Repeat on all your nails, let them dry, and apply your favorite clear topcoat for a finished look with multiple personalities: half glam girl and half rockabilly rager. Rawr!

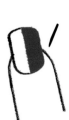

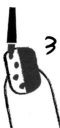

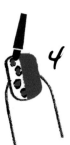

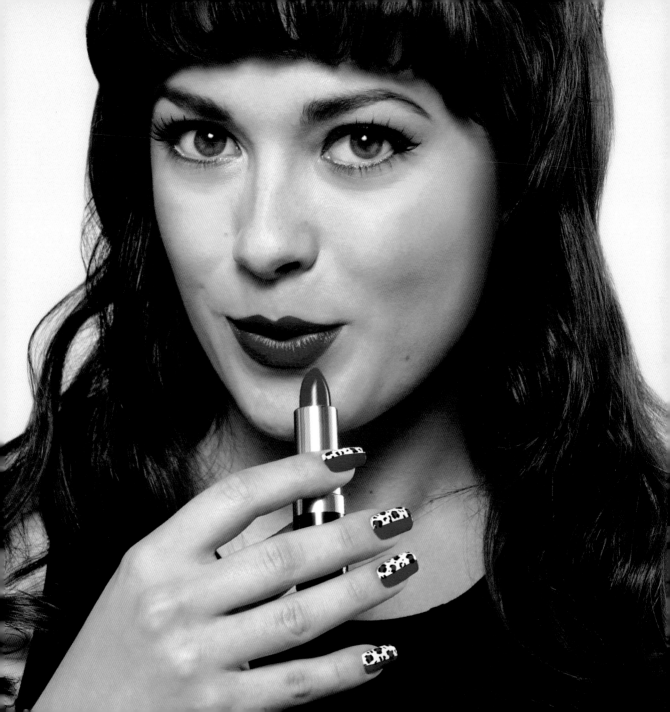

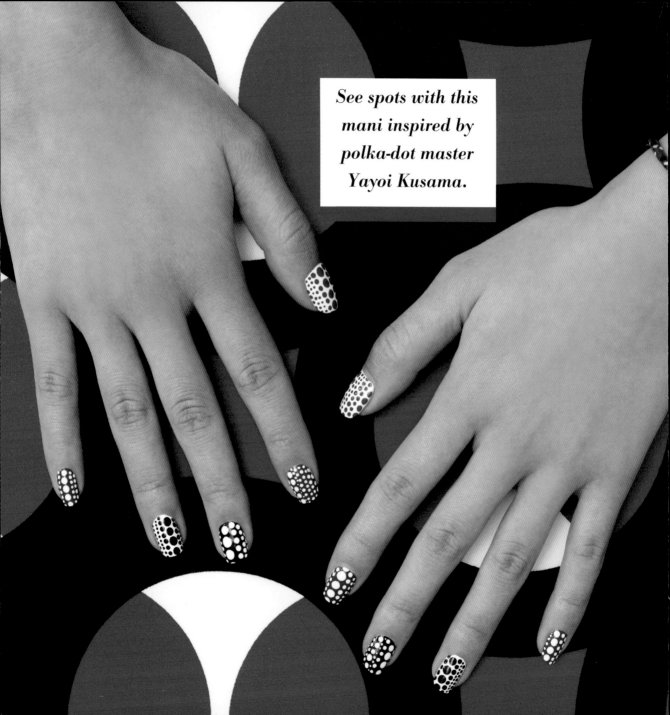

See spots with this mani inspired by polka-dot master Yayoi Kusama.

POP ON PLAYFUL
Polka Dots

STEP 1 ABC (apply basecoat), let it dry, and then paint each nail in one of three polish colors. Here we went white on thumbs and ring fingers, red on index fingers and pinkies, and black on middle fingers, but feel free to get creative with your color scheme and to invert your base and dot colors. Give your nails time to dry.

STEP 2 Pour white polish onto a piece of aluminum foil, then dip your largest dotting tool into it. Lightly dab the tool onto the red and black nails, using even pressure, to create vertical rows of dots.

STEP 3 Use a smaller dotting tool and the same polish to make vertical rows of dots next to the larger ones.

STEP 4 Repeat this process, switching up your dotting tool size, until your nails are covered in lines of dots. You can swap out the contrast, too—try black over white (like we do here on our ring fingers), red over white (like on our thumbs), and so on.

STEP 5 Let your dots dry, slick on a clear topcoat, and start spreading the whimsy.

MATERIALS

BASECOAT

WHITE, RED & BLACK POLISH

ALUMINUM FOIL

DOTTING TOOLS IN THREE SIZES

CLEAR TOPCOAT

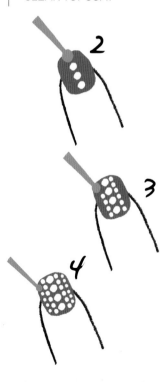

SAIL INTO THE SEASON WITH

Lots of Knots

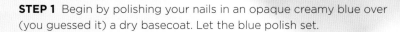

MATERIALS

BASECOAT

BLUE, BLACK & YELLOW POLISH

ALUMINUM FOIL

SMALL, ROUND PAINTBRUSH

CLEAR TOPCOAT

22 SILVER STUDS

DOTTING TOOL

STEP 1 Begin by polishing your nails in an opaque creamy blue over (you guessed it) a dry basecoat. Let the blue polish set.

STEP 2 Puddle black polish onto a piece of aluminum foil. With a small, round paintbrush, paint one connecting black swipe across your nails, curving or looping like a piece of rope. You won't be sorry if you plan your look before getting your nails involved—think about which nails get a loop, which you want to sparkle, and how each nail's rope design will link up when your fingers are side by side.

STEP 3 Rinse your paintbrush, then spill some yellow polish onto your foil palette. Paint tiny yellow diagonal lines inside each black swipe, leaving a small space between each yellow line. Let dry.

STEP 4 Apply a thin layer of topcoat. Hot tip: Your topcoat will help to smooth out brushstrokes in your primary color, flattening them into an even surface, so don't skip this step!

STEP 5 To add an anchor on your accent nails, first arrange your studs into the shape on a flat surface so you'll be able to place them onto your nails easily.

STEP 6 Apply a second layer of topcoat to your first accent nail. Dip your dotting tool in topcoat and use it to pick up a stud and place it on the nail. Repeat with half your studs, pressing them onto the nail, and then dazzle up your other accent nail, too.

STEP 7 Finish with a final layer of clear topcoat over your accent nails. Did someone say, "Anchors aweigh!"?

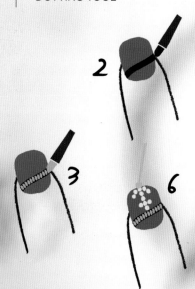

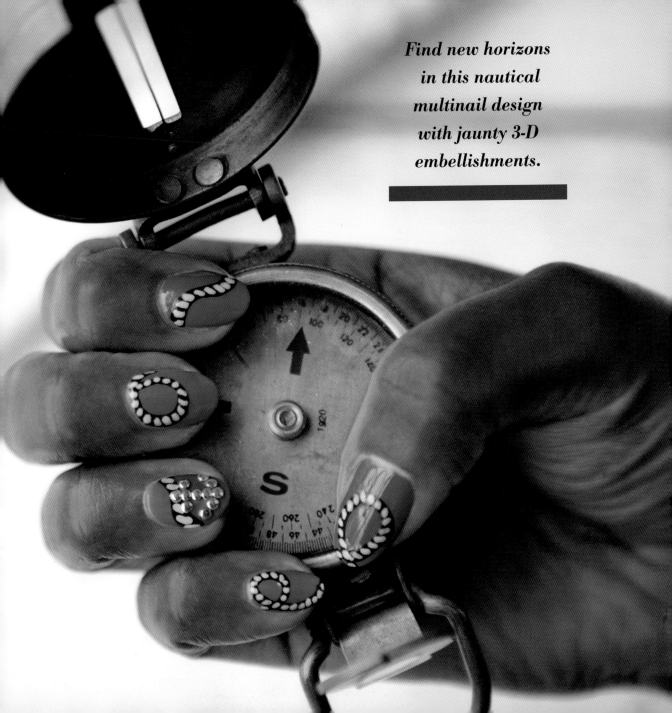

Find new horizons in this nautical multinail design with jauny 3-D embellishments.

BUTTON UP IN *Tiny Tuxes*

STEP 1 Mani it up with a glittery blue polish over your dry basecoat.

STEP 2 After your nails dry, pour white polish on some aluminum foil. Dip a striping brush in it and paint a deep V shape across the top half of your middle fingernail. Then fill in the V for a tuxedo-shirt effect.

STEP 3 Use the striping brush and the white polish to create the outlines of the collar, just outside the shirt.

STEP 4 When your nail is dry, add a drop of your black polish to the foil. Pick up a little with the dotting tool and make three or four button dots.

STEP 5 Finally, add some red polish to the foil. Dip your small, round paintbrush in and make two triangles at the widest part of the tuxedo shirt's white V.

STEP 6 Repeat on your other middle finger (and on any other nails you want to dress up!). Then let your tuxes dry and lock this dandy mani down with a clear topcoat.

MATERIALS

BASECOAT

BLUE GLITTER, WHITE, BLACK & RED POLISH

ALUMINUM FOIL

STRIPING BRUSH

DOTTING TOOL

SMALL, ROUND PAINTBRUSH

CLEAR TOPCOAT

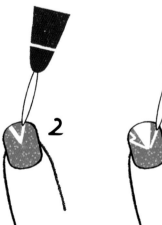
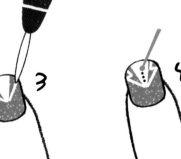
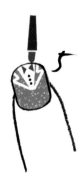

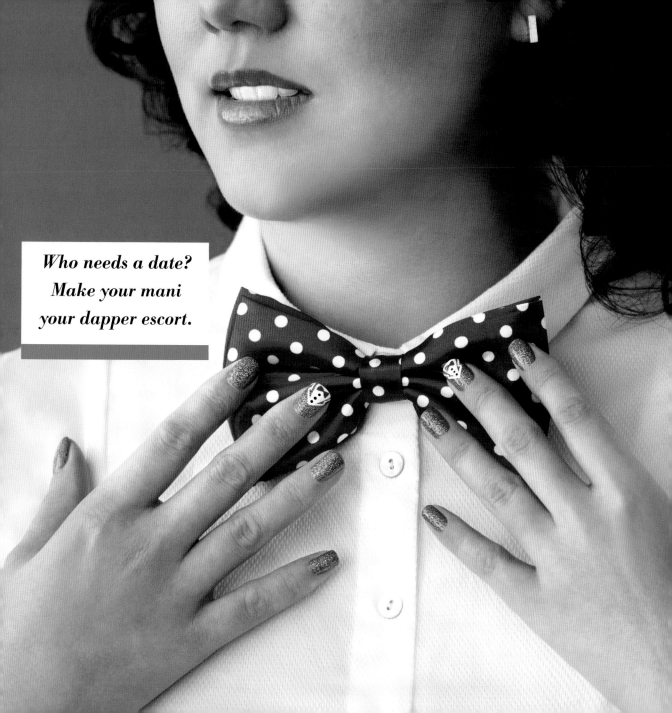

Who needs a date?
Make your mani
your dapper escort.

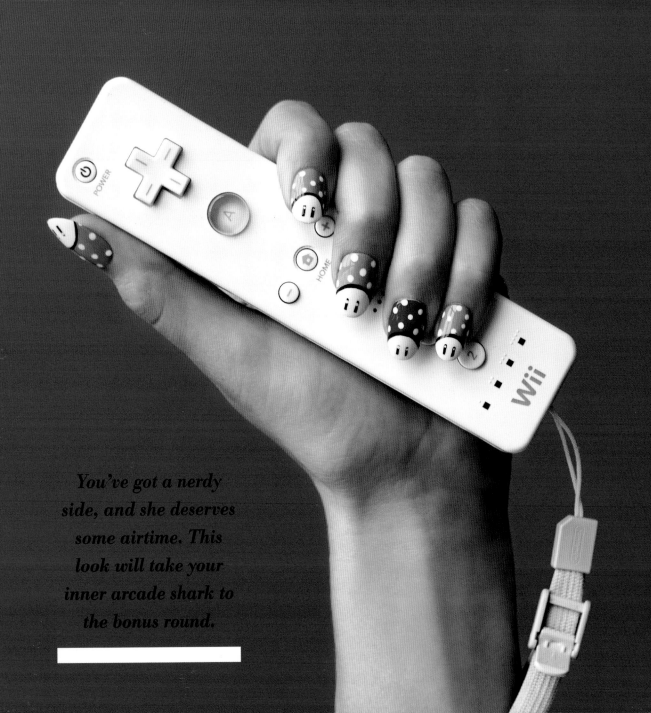

You've got a nerdy
side, and she deserves
some airtime. This
look will take your
inner arcade shark to
the bonus round.

UNLEASH YOUR GEEK ON A 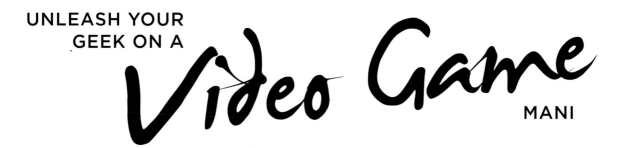Video Game MANI

STEP 1 Apply your basecoat, let it dry, then paint your nails with green and red polish and let them dry again. We love the quirky contrast of going green on everything but your red ring finger.

STEP 2 Grab your white polish and use the tip of its bottle brush to create a half-moon at each nail's free edge. To do this, place the brush in the middle of the nail and swoop it toward one side. Then refresh the paint and repeat the swoop on the other side.

STEP 3 Once your white tips are dry, load your striping brush with black polish and paint an outline around the white crescent on each nail.

STEP 4 Pour white polish onto your trusty aluminum foil palette. With the larger dotting tool, speckle your colored mushroom tops with white dots.

STEP 5 To make the eyes of the mushroom, use your striping brush to paint two even black stripes in the center of each white crescent.

STEP 6 After these black stripes dry, use your smaller dotting tool to place a white dot near one end of each black stripe.

STEP 7 Once your nails are totally dry, brush on a layer of clear topcoat. Unpause the game and grab the controls with confidence!

MATERIALS

BASECOAT

GREEN, RED, WHITE & BLACK POLISH

STRIPING BRUSH

ALUMINUM FOIL

DOTTING TOOLS IN TWO SIZES

CLEAR TOPCOAT

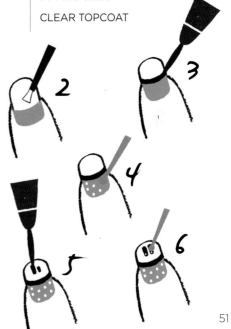

51

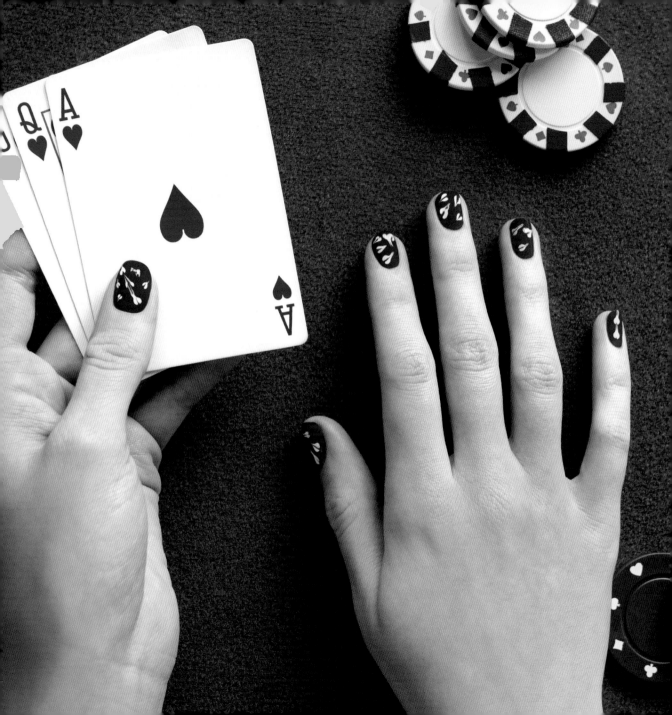

Pierce Hearts

WITH A NEEDLEPOINT MANI

MATERIALS

BASECOAT

DEEP RED & WHITE POLISH

NEEDLE

CLEAR TOPCOAT

STEP 1 Start with a dry basecoat and a basic mani in a sensual red. Wait for this coat to dry completely.

STEP 2 Paint a second coat of your base color onto your first nail. Immediately drip droplets of white polish where you want hearts to be, but don't stress about making them even—this style is all about a loose, relaxed pattern.

STEP 3 While the nail is still wet, gently place your needle or pin into a white polish droplet, and drag it to create your desired design. Be careful not to insert the needle too far—it shouldn't go through your first coat of polish.

STEP 4 Repeat this process until your nails are covered with tiny, adorable hearts, switching up the direction in which you pull the needle for a more dynamic array.

STEP 5 Let your nails dry, then seal your valentines with a clear topcoat.

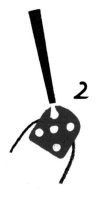

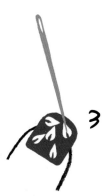

It's like that foam heart the cute barista puts on your latte, only it's for your nails.

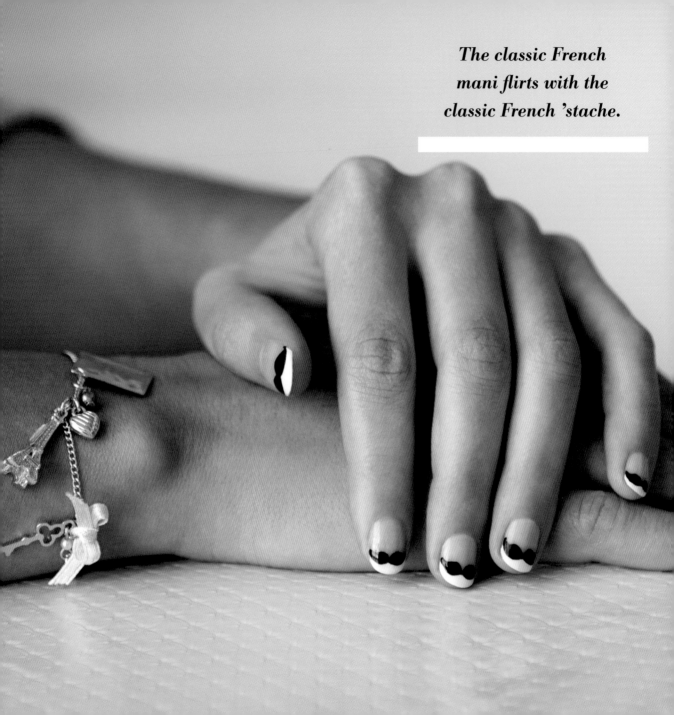

The classic French mani flirts with the classic French 'stache.

DON SOME Dainty Mustaches

MATERIALS

CLEAR BASECOAT

ADHESIVE BANDAGE

WHITE & BLACK POLISH

ALUMINUM FOIL

DOTTING TOOLS IN TWO SIZES

SMALL, ROUND PAINTBRUSH

CLEAR TOPCOAT

STEP 1 Start with a clear basecoat. Once it's dry, peel off the back of an adhesive bandage and press the bandage onto your first nail so that just the white nail edge is exposed. Swipe white polish over the exposed tip and remove your bandage; repeat this process on all your nails. Voilà! Stop here and you have a classic French mani.

STEP 2 To make mustaches, drop a dollop of black polish onto a piece of aluminum foil. When your tips are dry, use the larger dotting tool to pick up a small amount of black polish and make two dots, barely touching, where the clear and white polish meet on each nail.

STEP 3 Grab more polish with the smaller dotting tool and make small dots on either side of the two larger circles. These small dots will form the mustaches' tips.

STEP 4 Dip your small, round paintbrush into the black polish, then connect the smaller dots to the larger ones with symmetrical swoops.

STEP 5 After your nails dry, finish your set of mini 'staches with clear topcoat. Facial hair never looked so femme-fabulous.

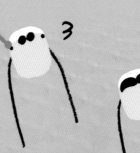

Half-Moons

STEP 1 Over your dry basecoat, paint your nails the color you'd like in the moon area—that's the little semicircle above your cuticles, aptly called the lunula. We used white. Apply two coats and let them dry.

STEP 2 Use the hole-punch protectors to cover a half-circle at the base of each nail, overlapping onto the skin. If a sticker is stiff and not lying flat, cut a slit in one side (just make sure you cut into the sticker where it touches your skin, not your nail) and overlap the two edges.

STEP 3 Carefully paint the second color (in our mani, that's black) over the protector's edge and up through the tip of each nail. Cue up a classic movie while you let this coat dry, then repeat with a second.

STEP 4 Slowly peel off each sticker, revealing the white half-moon underneath.

STEP 5 This look may get its graphic grace from posh art deco stylings, but that doesn't mean you can't edge it out. Carefully paint the undersides of your nails in a surprising shade, like this flashy lime green.

STEP 6 Seal the deal with a clear topcoat.

MATERIALS

BASECOAT

WHITE, BLACK & LIME GREEN POLISH

HOLE-PUNCH PROTECTORS

CLEAR TOPCOAT

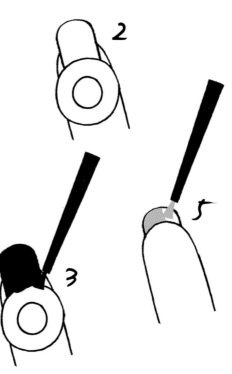

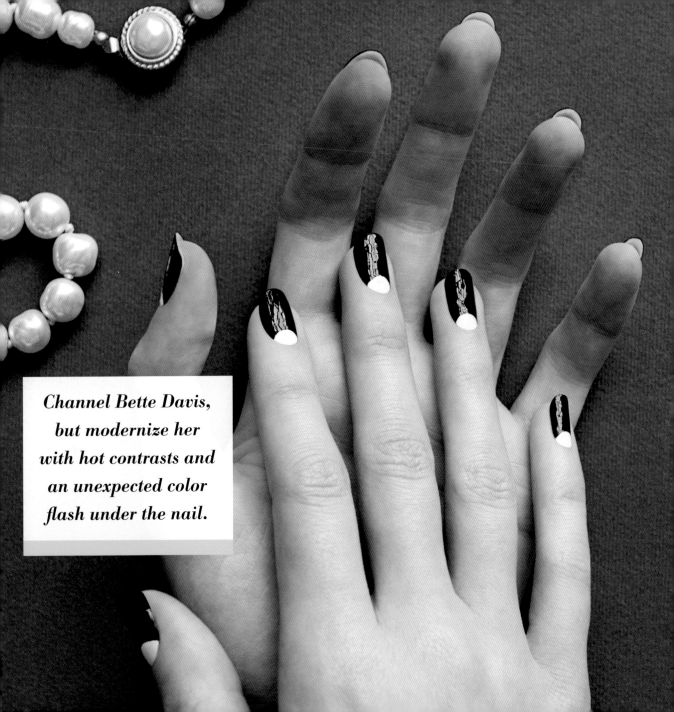

Channel Bette Davis, but modernize her with hot contrasts and an unexpected color flash under the nail.

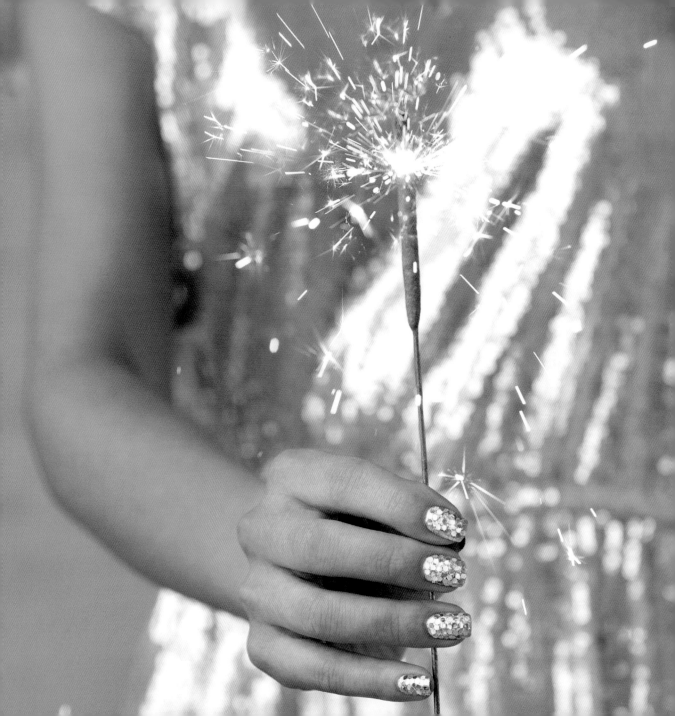

LIGHT UP THE NIGHT IN

Mirror Ball

NAILS

MATERIALS

BASECOAT

SILVER METALLIC FOIL POLISH

CLEAR TOPCOAT

ALUMINUM FOIL

DOTTING TOOL

LARGE HEXAGONAL SILVER GLITTER

STEP 1 Don't forget to ABC (apply basecoat) and let it dry. Then kick things off with a basic manicure in a silver metallic foil polish.

STEP 2 Let your nails dry, then place a large drop of clear topcoat on an aluminum foil palette. Use your dotting tool to pick up some topcoat and make a large dot on your first nail.

STEP 3 Use the same tool to pick up a piece of hexagonal glitter and press it into the topcoat.

STEP 4 Continue placing glitter pieces until the nail is fully covered with glitter. For optimal coverage, line up the edges of each glitter piece, and cut a few pieces to fill any gaps where your nail meets the cuticle or sidewall. It's been our experience that no amount of glitter is ever too much, in life as in this manicure.

STEP 5 Repeat on all your nails until your fingers are glinting like disco balls. Finish with clear topcoat. Now there's nothing to do but dance!

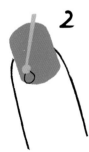

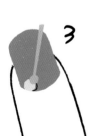

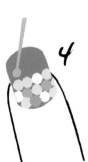

This style takes time, but the results are blindingly brilliant. Let sparkles fly!

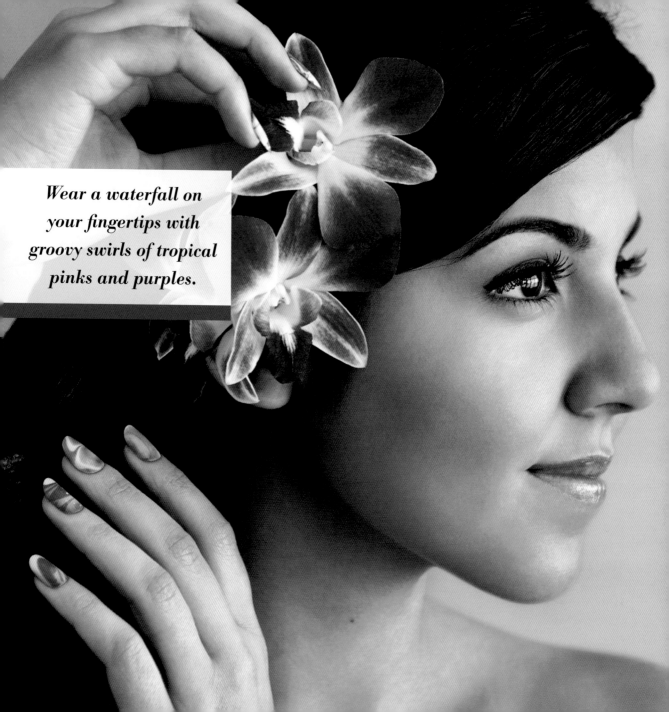

Wear a waterfall on your fingertips with groovy swirls of tropical pinks and purples.

DIP YOUR 'TIPS FOR
Marbled Magic

STEP 1 Start with a dry layer of basecoat, then lacquer your nails in a light pink polish to make your marbling vivid. In this trick (which we've borrowed from old-school artists), you create a pattern by blending colors on the water's surface, then pressing your canvas—in this case, your nail—on the surface of the water to pick up the design.

STEP 2 This process can get messy! While the polish dries, put tape on the skin surrounding your nails to keep it clear of excess polish.

STEP 3 Fill your glass two-thirds full with water. Load up the brush of your first color—here, we used lilac—and let a big drop fall gently into the liquid. Continue with your other colors—white, followed by purple—until you have several concentric rings of polish on the water's surface.

STEP 4 Drag a toothpick through the polish rings, starting at the outside and pulling toward the center of the glass. Continue dragging, trying crisscrosses, diamond shapes, and big and little swirls, until you're a fan of what you see.

STEP 5 Gently plunge a fingernail into the glass, submerging the nail. Crucial hot tip: Make sure the nail plate makes horizontal contact with the water's surface—don't dunk your fingertip vertically in the water.

STEP 6 Holding your nail on the water's surface, use the toothpick to trace around your fingertip, breaking up the extra polish on the water's surface without disturbing the polish directly under the nail.

STEP 7 Lift your finger out of the water and let it dry before removing your tape. Repeat the drop-drag-dip process on all your nails. When all the tape is off, fill a dappen dish with acetone and use an angled brush to clean up around the edges.

STEP 8 Seal in your marbled swirls with clear topcoat.

MATERIALS

BASECOAT

LIGHT PINK, LILAC, WHITE & PURPLE POLISH

TAPE

SMALL GLASS OR CUP

ROOM TEMPERATURE BOTTLED WATER

TOOTHPICK

DAPPEN DISH

ACETONE

ANGLED BRUSH

CLEAR TOPCOAT

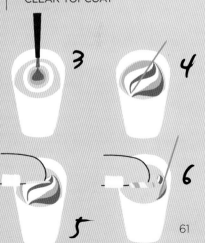

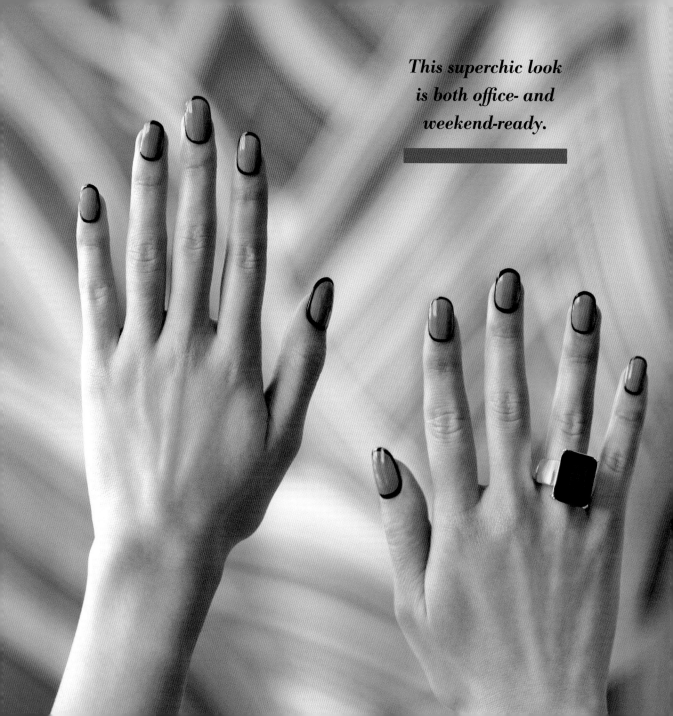

This superchic look is both office- and weekend-ready.

Outline

FOR IMPACT

MATERIALS

- BASECOAT
- SMALL, ROUND PAINTBRUSH
- BLACK & PURPLE POLISH
- ANGLED BRUSH
- DAPPEN DISH
- ACETONE
- CLEAR TOPCOAT

STEP 1 Apply a basecoat to your nails. Let it dry.

STEP 2 Dip your small, round paintbrush into your black polish and create a thin outline stripe around each nail's perimeter. Don't worry—this line doesn't have to be perfect since you'll cover the edges with your purple polish.

STEP 3 Let your black outlines dry, then rinse your brush and, starting near the cuticle, use it to make a crisp edge with purple polish inside the black outline. It's okay to overlap the black inside edge so it looks nice and clean.

STEP 4 Fill in the center of each nail with purple. Apply a second coat if you prefer a fully saturated color wash.

STEP 5 While your look dries, use an angled brush dipped in acetone to clean up any messes around the cuticle and skin—this is one look that begs for a tidy line. Top it all off with a clear topcoat, and you'll be megamod for days.

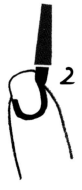
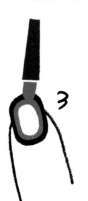
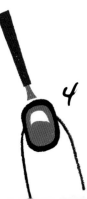

MAKE MINI
Monster MOUTHS

STEP 1 Lacquer each nail with hot pink nail polish over a dry basecoat. Let the pink polish dry, too.

STEP 2 Use the black polish's bottle brush to paint a curved line about one-quarter of the way above the base of each fingernail and another curved line about one-quarter of the way below the free edge, as if you're painting a black eye in the middle of your nail. Fill the area between the lines with black polish and let dry.

STEP 3 Pour white polish on some aluminum foil. Dip a small, round paintbrush into it and outline four fang shapes on each nail where the pink and black polish meet, pointing inward. Fill them in with white polish.

STEP 4 Add small white teeth until all your monster mouths have a full grill. Give these teeth a chance to dry.

STEP 5 To clean up any rough edges, dip a striping brush in a bottle of pink polish and add a strip of pink across the area where the pink and black polishes meet, overlapping the teeth to make a clean gum line.

STEP 6 Let your nails dry, then add a layer of clear topcoat. Get ready to bare your teeth everywhere!

MATERIALS

BASECOAT

HOT PINK, BLACK & WHITE POLISH

ALUMINUM FOIL

SMALL, ROUND PAINTBRUSH

STRIPING BRUSH

CLEAR TOPCOAT

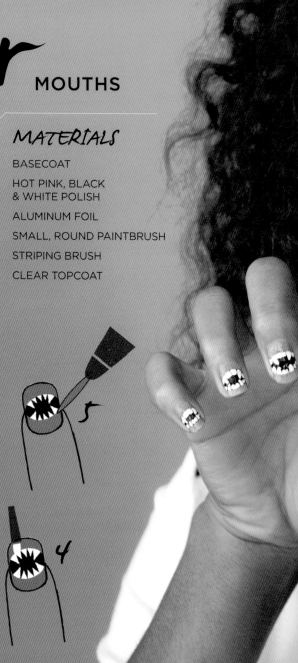

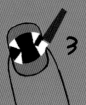

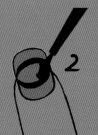

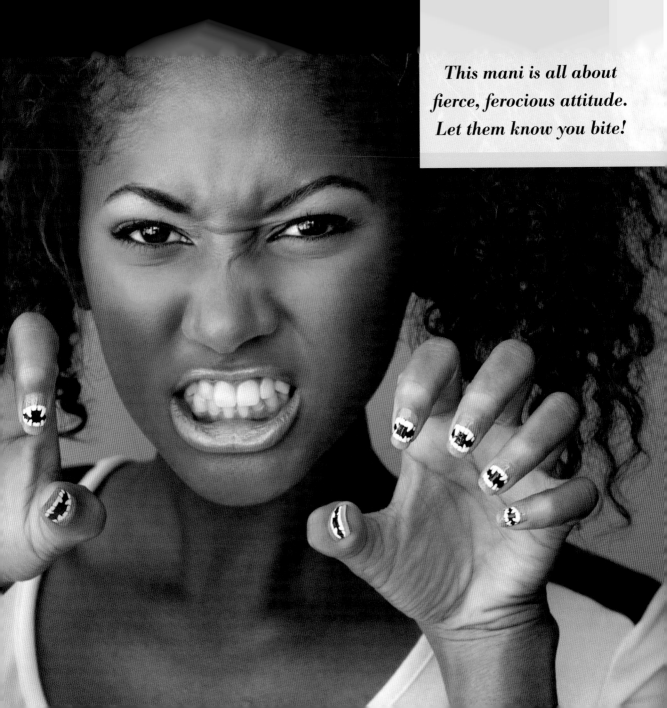

This mani is all about
fierce, ferocious attitude.
Let them know you bite!

FLASH FLORAL FINGERS IN A

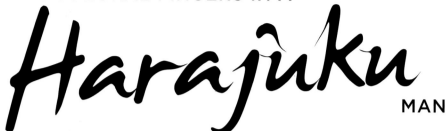

Harajuku MANI

STEP 1 Start by painting your nails with pastel pink polish over your dry basecoat. Let this dry.

STEP 2 Add darker pink, white, and tan polish to a piece of aluminum foil. Pick up dabs of these colors with a cosmetic sponge and splotch them onto your nails. Let this dry. Then add glitter polish to your foil, and sponge on a few sparkly patches of that, too.

STEP 3 Lay out your embellishments on a flat surface and scheme up your design (floral bouquets, lines, clusters, or whatever your heart desires). It'll make this over-the-top mani go much faster if you plan ahead, trust us.

STEP 4 After your polish is dry and your design is set, brush clear topcoat onto the first nail. Lightly touch a dotting tool against the clear topcoat, then use it to pick up an embellishment and press it into the topcoat, making sure each edge sticks in place. Add embellishments until the nail is so cute you almost can't take it anymore.

STEP 5 Repeat as desired on all your nails. You can leave some of the studs bare so they stand out, and paint over some with the first shade of pink polish for a coy monochrome look. (See how we painted the bow on our middle finger pink to make it blend in?) Let your nails dry.

STEP 6 Make it for keeps with a clear topcoat.

MATERIALS

BASECOAT

PASTEL PINK, DARKER PINK, WHITE & TAN POLISH

ALUMINUM FOIL

COSMETIC SPONGE

GLITTER POLISH

LOTS OF FLAT-BACKED EMBELLISHMENTS

CLEAR TOPCOAT

DOTTING TOOL

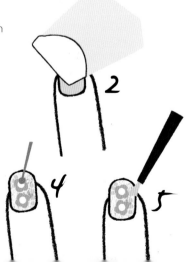

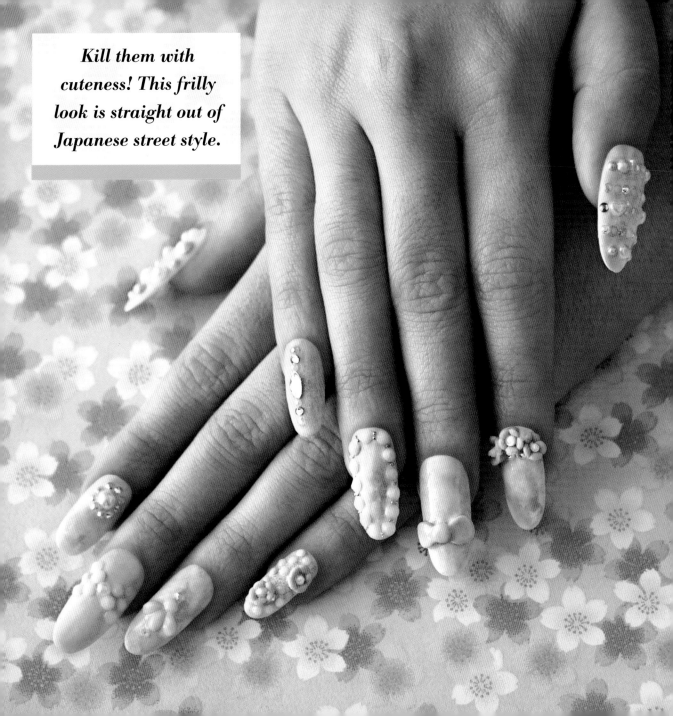

Kill them with cuteness! This frilly look is straight out of Japanese street style.

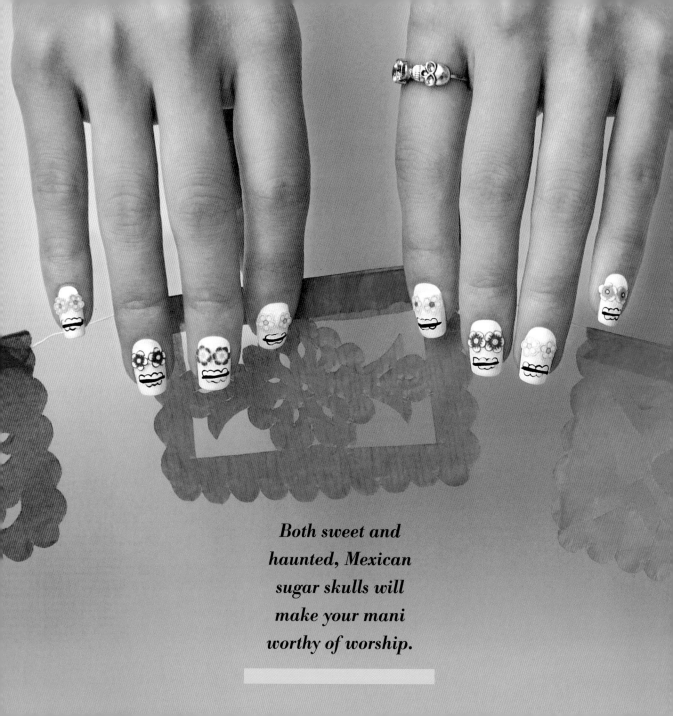

Both sweet and haunted, Mexican sugar skulls will make your mani worthy of worship.

SPIN SOME Sugar Skulls

FOR DÍA DE LOS MUERTOS

STEP 1 Start with your ABCs (apply basecoat) and let it dry. Then paint your fingernails with opaque white polish. The idea here is to play up your nail's natural skull shape to mimic those gleefully morbid crafts that are made by hand for Mexico's Day of the Dead celebration. Let your nails dry, then apply some clear topcoat and let that dry, too.

STEP 2 Place a dot of black polish onto the aluminum foil. Use your larger dotting tool to pick up some of the polish and make a row of dots in the center of each nail—these dots will form your skull's distinctive, grim little grin. Place another row of black dots just below this row. Let your dots dry.

STEP 3 Add some white polish to your foil palette and, with your smaller dotting tool, place white dots inside of the black dots you just made.

STEP 4 Once the teeth have dried completely, dip your striping brush in black polish and paint a narrow black line through the center of your skull's mouth on each nail. Let these dry.

STEP 5 The trick to this look's majorly festive 3-D appeal? Fimo flowers—accents made of pliable clay—that you can scoop up at a beauty-supply store near you. To apply them, start with a layer of clear topcoat, then touch your large dotting tool to the topcoat and use it to push a flower onto a nail. Really press it on there, then add a second to form a pair of eyes. Repeat on each nail.

STEP 6 Carefully apply another layer of topcoat over each nail to preserve those skulls for posterity! Light a candle as you reflect on the past in a mani that's all about the now.

MATERIALS

- BASECOAT
- WHITE & BLACK POLISH
- CLEAR TOPCOAT
- ALUMINUM FOIL
- DOTTING TOOLS IN TWO SIZES
- STRIPING BRUSH
- 20 FIMO FLOWERS

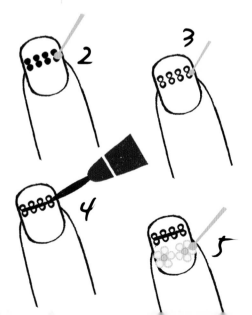

69

HEAT UP THE STREETS IN A
Haute Couture
MANI

MATERIALS

STRIPING TAPE

SCISSORS

BASECOAT

BLACK POLISH

CLEAR TOPCOAT

MATTE TOPCOAT

TWEEZERS

FINE GOLD CHAIN

NAIL GLUE

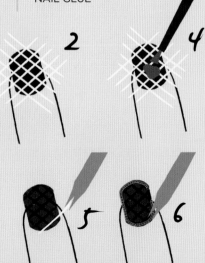

STEP 1 Cut striping tape into 100 narrow strips a little longer than your nails, then paint your nails a shiny black over a dry basecoat. After they dry, slick on a thin layer of clear topcoat and let that dry, too.

STEP 2 Apply criss-crossing strips of tape diagonally so that they create networks of diamond shapes on each nail. Press that tape down tight—no polish leaks!

STEP 3 Apply a thin coat of your black polish, covering the tape. Repeat with another thin coat, letting each dry between applications. Hot tip: The more layers you slather on, the more quilted your nails will look.

STEP 4 Apply a thin layer of fast-drying clear topcoat to all your nails. Once that's dry, apply matte topcoat, too.

STEP 5 Wait until your nails are completely dry (really, we mean it—it may take up to an hour for the layers to set, which is why it's great to do this look on a set of nail tips) before slowly, carefully peeling off the tape with tweezers.

STEP 6 Using scissors, cut enough gold chain to wrap around one of your nails. Trace nail glue around the edge of your chosen nail, then lay the chain over the topcoat using tweezers, pressing it down a little at a time.

STEP 7 Repeat on your other hand's accent nail. No matter where you bought your bag, there's nothing faux about this glam accessory—this mani is the real deal.

70

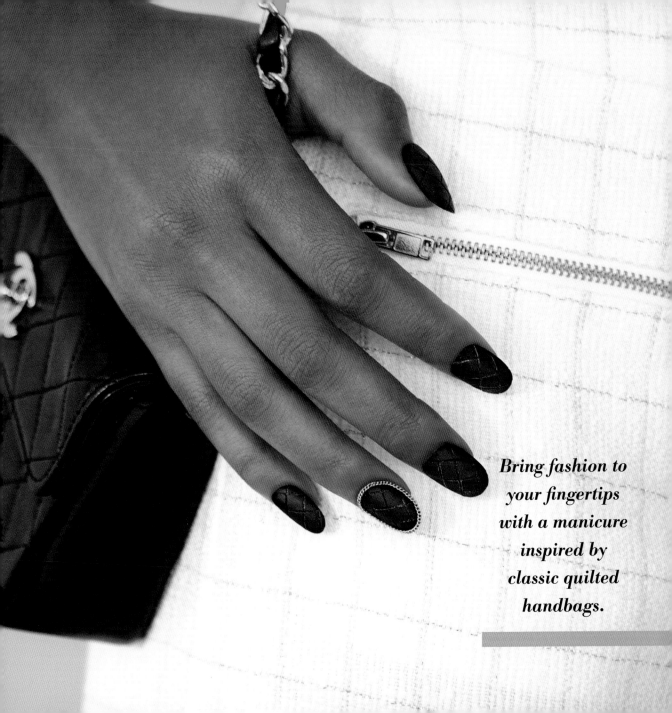

Bring fashion to your fingertips with a manicure inspired by classic quilted handbags.

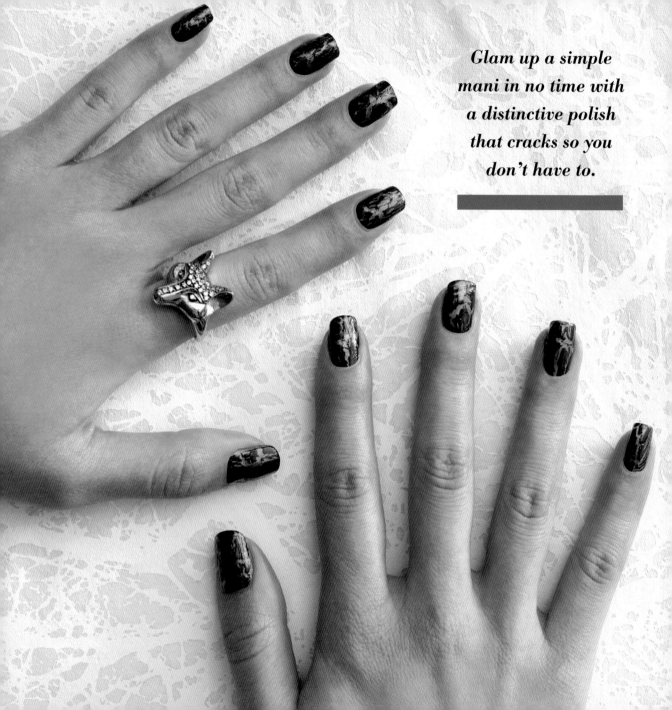

Glam up a simple mani in no time with a distinctive polish that cracks so you don't have to.

SNAP, CRACKLE &

Pop a Topcoat

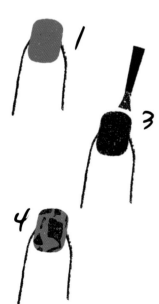

MATERIALS

BASECOAT

EMERALD POLISH

BLACK CRACKLE
TOPCOAT

CLEAR TOPCOAT

STEP 1 Paint each nail with a color you love over a dry basecoat. We're nutty for this emerald green, but a hot pink, electric blue, or glowing yellow would look foxy, too.

STEP 2 While your nails are drying, give a good think to what sort of crackle effect you're after. The crackles follow the brushstrokes, so the way you paint with this specialized polish will create different results. The thinner the coat, the more fine and straight your lines will be, while a thicker coat will yield larger polish pieces with wide cracks—for this effect, don't apply much pressure to the brush.

STEP 3 Once your nails are dry, layer on your crackle topcoat. Alternate painting on the crackle polish horizontally and diagonally for dynamic gaps and gashes.

STEP 4 Make sure to work quickly—these polishes dry fast. Don't brush another layer over wet crackle or it won't break! Instead, wait and watch the polish magically shatter, revealing the base color underneath. The beauty of this mani's look is that the polish does all the hard work for you.

STEP 5 Once your crackle is dry, protect your work with a clear topcoat. Snap and Pop have never been more jealous.

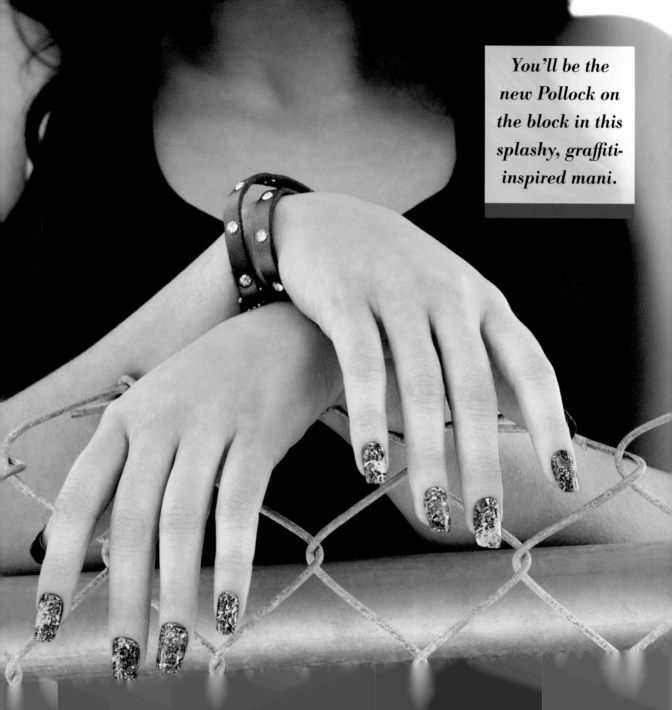

You'll be the new Pollock on the block in this splashy, graffiti-inspired mani.

TAG YOUR 'TIPS WITH

Splatter Paint

MATERIALS

BASECOAT

BLACK, GRAY & HOT PINK POLISH

TAPE

SKINNY COCKTAIL STRAWS

ANGLED BRUSH

DAPPEN DISH

ACETONE

CLEAR TOPCOAT

STEP 1 Give yourself a black mani over a dry basecoat. Protect the skin around your nails with tape. Or, if you're living on the edge, skip the tape and clean up bloopers later.

STEP 2 After your black polish dries, dip the tip of the gray polish brush onto the end of a cocktail straw so that the bottom end of the straw fills up with a small amount of polish. Place your finger over the top end to create suction so the polish doesn't drip out.

STEP 3 Hold the polish-filled end of the straw above your nails. Place your mouth on the straw's other end and quickly blow through it to launch gray polish onto your nails. (Hot tip: Don't inhale.) Keep blowing paint onto all of your nails.

STEP 4 When your gray splatters are dry, repeat the blowing process on all your nails with hot pink polish (and any other colors you like). Remove the tape and tidy up any stray splatters with an angled brush dipped in a dish of acetone.

STEP 5 After your splattered paint job dries, seal it in with clear topcoat and give your mani masterpiece a highbrow title like *Spicy Splatter #3*. You've arrived!

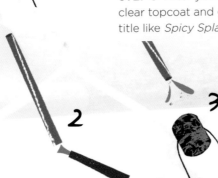

2

3

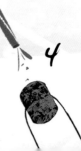

4

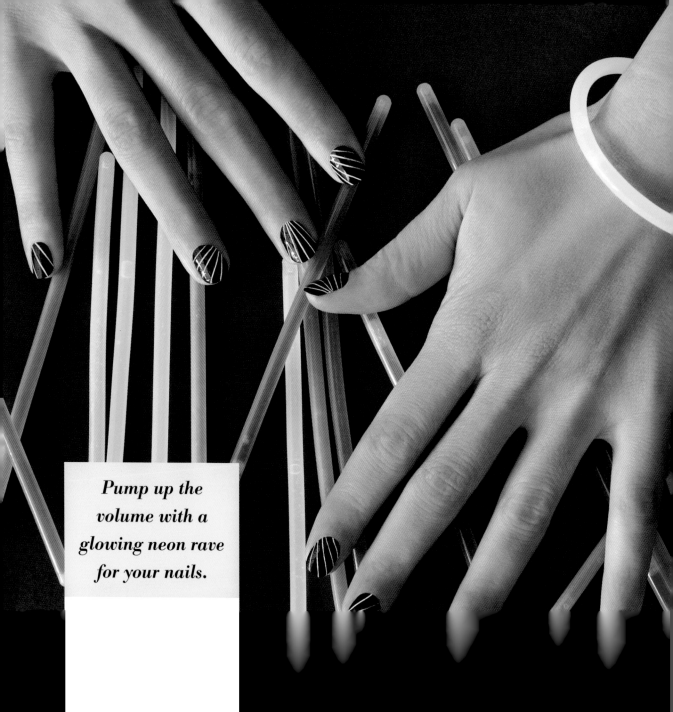

Pump up the volume with a glowing neon rave for your nails.

SHINE A
Laser Show

STEP 1 Cut striping tape into pieces a little longer than your nails. You'll need about fifty strips for a full manicure.

STEP 2 Manicure your nails with a basecoat, let it dry, and follow with an opaque white shade. (The white polish will make those neon colors really scream.) Let your nails dry again.

STEP 3 Add a drop of your first neon shade to a piece of aluminum foil and pick up a small amount with your cosmetic sponge's tip. Dab the sponge over your nails to randomly distribute polish. Repeat with your other hues, adding extra coats for a more intense effect. What you want are zones of color fading into each other with a soft edge. Let your nails dry.

STEP 4 Press striping tape onto your nails in a starburst shape. (It's cool to let the tape extend past the nails' edges.) We mixed up the angle of the laser beams for some rave-tastic variety.

STEP 5 Make sure all pieces of tape are pressed down firmly, then coat your nails with two layers of black polish, letting them dry between applications.

STEP 6 When your nails are dry, remove each piece of striping tape by grasping one end with your tweezers and peeling it off.

STEP 7 Apply a layer of clear topcoat. Let the dance party begin.

MATERIALS

STRIPING TAPE

SCISSORS

BASECOAT

WHITE, PINK, YELLOW, GREEN, ORANGE & BLACK POLISH

ALUMINUM FOIL

COSMETIC SPONGE

TWEEZERS

CLEAR TOPCOAT

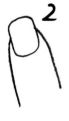
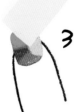
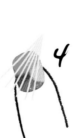
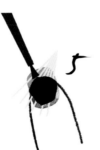

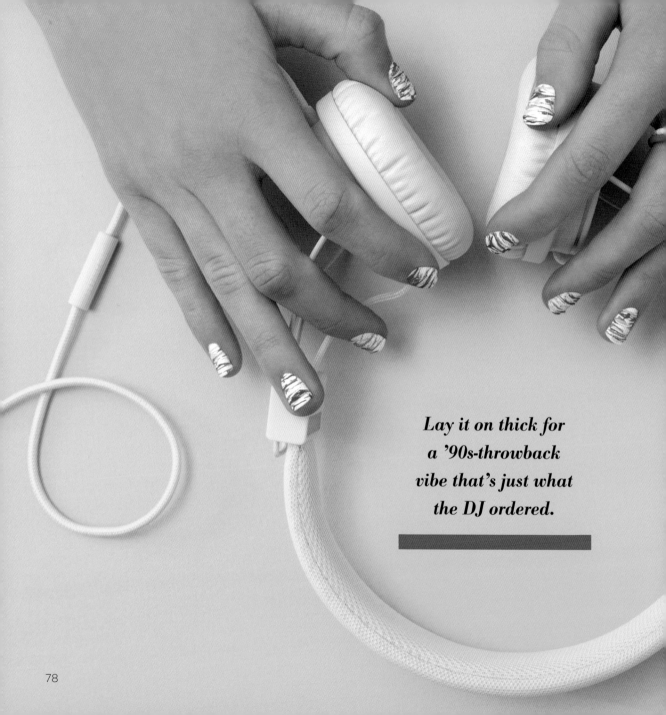

Lay it on thick for
a '90s-throwback
vibe that's just what
the DJ ordered.

Puff-Paint

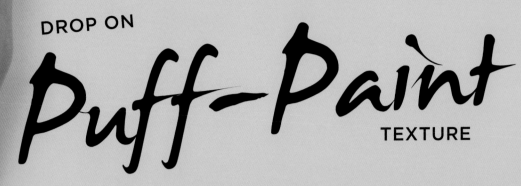

TEXTURE

MATERIALS

BASECOAT

WHITE, NEON YELLOW, BRIGHT GREEN, HOT PINK & TANGERINE POLISH

CLEAR TOPCOAT

ALUMINUM FOIL

TOOTHPICK

STEP 1 Start with a basecoat, let it dry, and then slather on an opaque white. When that's dry, slick on a clear topcoat.

STEP 2 The key to this mani is patience! After your clear topcoat dries, pour a large pool of yellow polish on a piece of aluminum foil and wait for it to thicken up as it starts to dry. Test the consistency by dipping your toothpick into the polish and lifting it out. If the toothpick pulls up a thick string of polish, you're good to go.

STEP 3 Pick up a small amount of stringy polish with the toothpick and wrap it over a fingertip, letting a thick thread of polish drop onto the nail. Drag polish two or three times across the first nail, then use that color on all your nails.

STEP 4 Repeat the process with the green, pink, and tangerine colors on all your nails until you've built up a rad variety of hues and textures. Who's got the boom box?

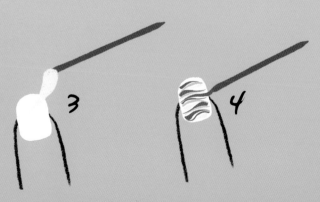

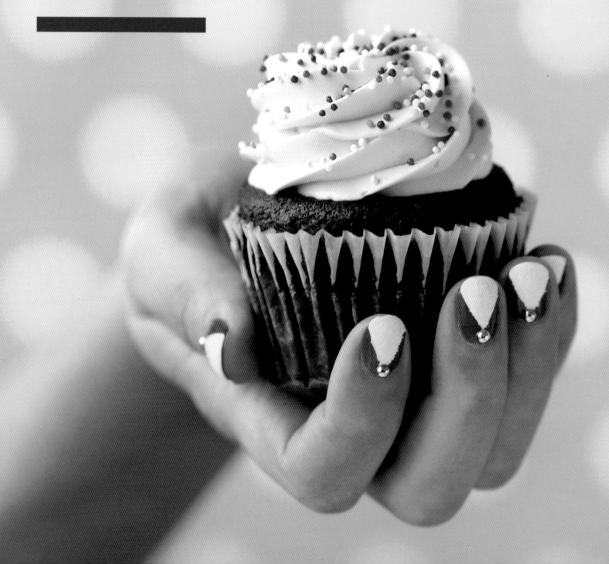

Flocking powder adds a luxe, tactile texture that makes nails look like a sweet treat.

Velvety Tips

MATERIALS

BASECOAT

BRIGHT PINK & WHITE POLISH

CLEAR TOPCOAT

TAPE

WHITE FLOCKING POWDER

DOTTING TOOL

10 FLAT-BACKED GOLD PEARLS

STEP 1 After ABCing (applying basecoat), let your nails dry and paint on a pink polish that will pop against white flocking powder, which is a fine talc that gives a felt-like finish. (You can pick up some at any good crafts-supply store near you!)

STEP 2 After your nails dry, give them a layer of clear topcoat and let them set. Then place two pieces of tape over one nail to create a V shape. Repeat this on all your nails.

STEP 3 Brush white polish inside the V shape and then immediately sprinkle it with flocking powder, using the cap with the smallest holes. Go ahead, paint your other nails with white and dust them, too.

STEP 4 Use a dotting tool to apply a dab of clear topcoat at the V shape's bottom, then use the dotting tool to press on a flat-backed gold pearl. Add pearls to your other nails and revel in your oh-so-touchable tips.

2

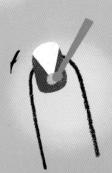

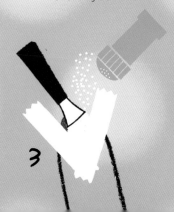

3

TIE TOGETHER
Pretty Bows

MATERIALS

BASECOAT

GRAY, BRIGHT PINK, LIGHT PINK, ROSE, YELLOW & WHITE POLISH

ALUMINUM FOIL

SMALL, ROUND PAINTBRUSH

DOTTING TOOL

CLEAR TOPCOAT

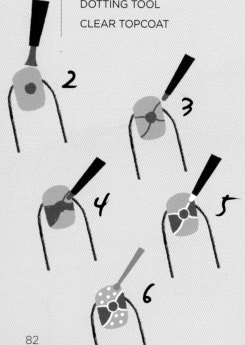

STEP 1 Start with a dry basecoat, then do a basic mani in a different adorable color on each nail. Let your nails dry.

STEP 2 Grab a color that contrasts nicely with your first nail's base color (we started with a bright pink bow over gray) and place a dot of it in the nail's center.

STEP 3 Dab some of the same polish on a piece of aluminum foil and load up your small, round paintbrush. Then paint two curved lines extending from each side of the center dot to the nail's sidewalls.

STEP 4 Fill in the areas on either side of your dot with polish, creating the bow's ribbon shape. Do a second coat if necessary for an evenly colored bow. Now that you've mastered this lovely little knot, branch out and make bows on the rest of your nails in all different colors, rinsing your brush between each shade. Let them dry.

STEP 5 Place some opaque white polish on the foil and, after rinsing the small paintbrush, use it to outline all your bows. Start by outlining the small circle in the middle, then trace the ribbon loops' edges.

STEP 6 Use a dotting tool to fill in the spaces around the bows with a silly smattering of polka dots.

STEP 7 When your bows are dry, sweep on a clear topcoat. See? Sweet 'n' easy.

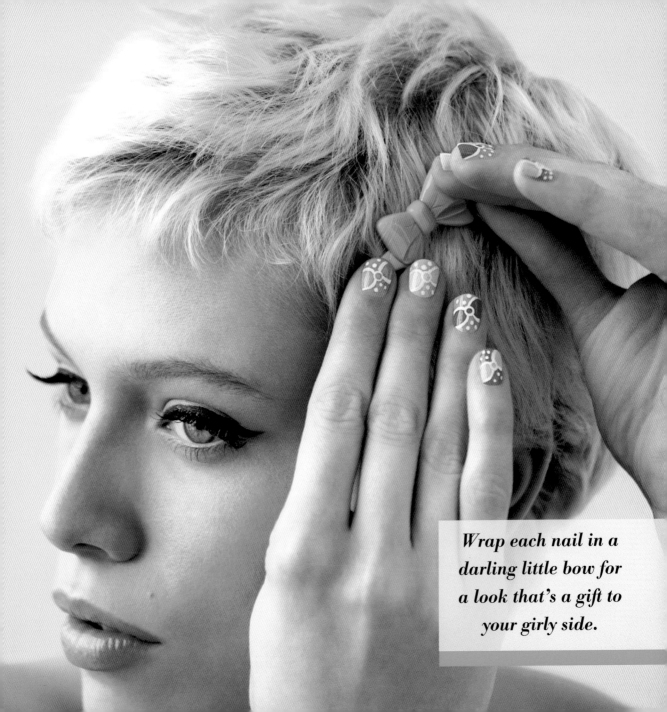

Wrap each nail in a darling little bow for a look that's a gift to your girly side.

Out-of-This-World

GALAXY NAILS

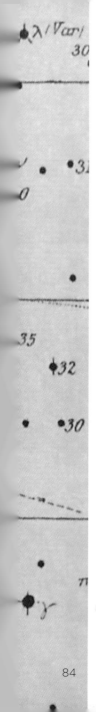

MATERIALS

BASECOAT

BLACK, WHITE, GREEN, BLUE, YELLOW & SILVER HOLOGRAPHIC GLITTER POLISH

ALUMINUM FOIL

COSMETIC SPONGE

DOTTING TOOL

CLEAR TOPCOAT

STEP 1 ABC (apply basecoat). Once the basecoat has set, do a basic manicure with black polish. Let your nails dry.

STEP 2 Pour white polish onto a piece of aluminum foil. Dip in the cosmetic sponge and dab white splotches across each nail. This will serve as a backdrop for brighter space dust particles, making them really visible against the black—even without a telescope. Let this dry.

STEP 3 Place a dollop of green polish on the foil, pick some up with the sponge, and dab it lightly over half of the white areas. For a realistic effect, try to minimize harsh outlines. Allow it to dry.

STEP 4 Sponge on blue polish using the same technique, but cover the second half of the white areas, blending the blue into the green.

STEP 5 When these layers are dry, lightly sponge silver holographic glitter polish over your nails for a shimmery, far-away starfield.

STEP 6 Dab a little yellow polish on the sponge. Press it onto the nebulae you've already created for more explosions of space dust.

STEP 7 To create the illusion of space's distance and depth, dip a dotting tool in white polish and scatter on a few larger, closer stars.

STEP 8 When your nails are dry, lock in your clear night sky with a glossy topcoat. You're ready for blastoff!

2

3

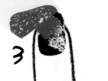

4

5

6

7

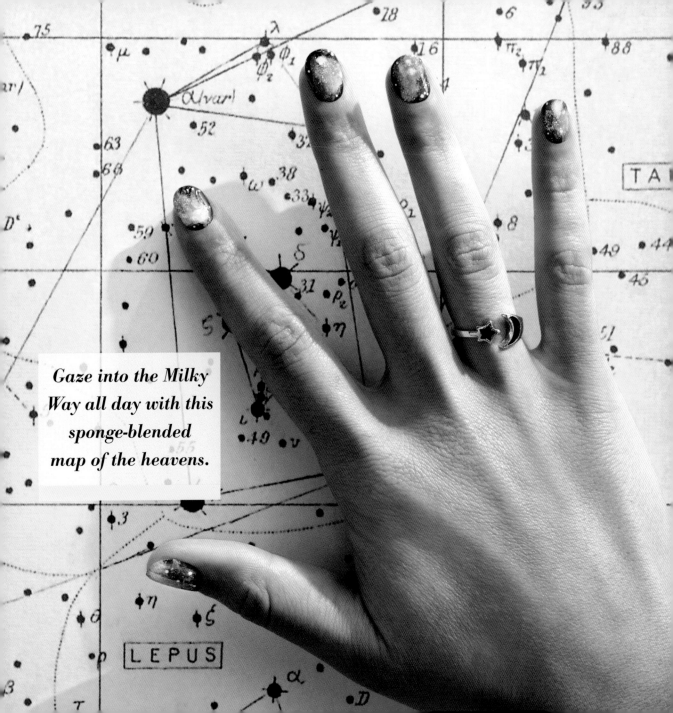

Gaze into the Milky Way all day with this sponge-blended map of the heavens.

LACE UP
Saucy Lingerie
NAILS

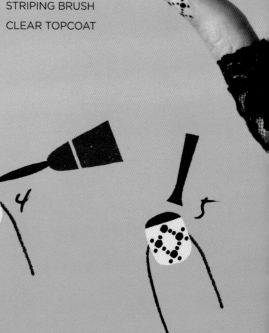

STEP 1 Start with a dry basecoat, then paint all your nails with a color that matches your skin tone.

STEP 2 When your mani is dry, add a bit of black polish to a piece of aluminum foil. Collect a drop of it with your larger dotting tool and place four dots on each nail to make a diamond shape.

STEP 3 Use the smaller dotting tool to add smaller dots between the larger dots, forming a sexy fishnet pattern.

STEP 4 Load a striping brush up with black polish and swipe it horizontally across the top of each nail to outline a French tip.

STEP 5 Dip the bottle brush in the black polish and use it to fill in your tip areas.

STEP 6 Let your nails dry and add a clear topcoat to prevent runs in these sassy stockings. Ooh la la!

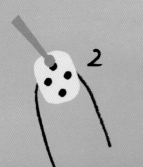

2

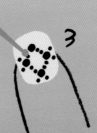

3

4

5

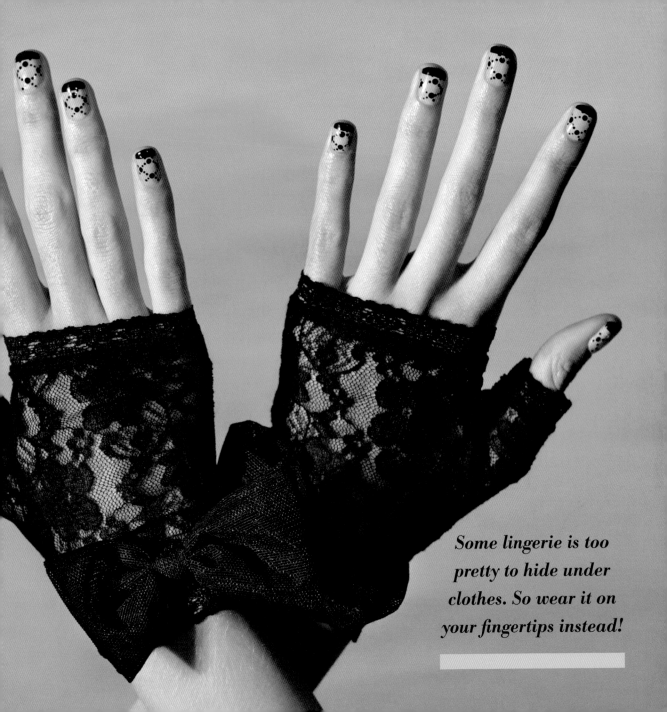

Some lingerie is too pretty to hide under clothes. So wear it on your fingertips instead!

LIVE LA VIE BOHÈME IN AN *Ikat* STYLE

MATERIALS

BASECOAT

PALE BLUE, BLACK, DEEP PINK & WHITE POLISH

ALUMINUM FOIL

SMALL, ROUND PAINTBRUSH

CLEAR TOPCOAT

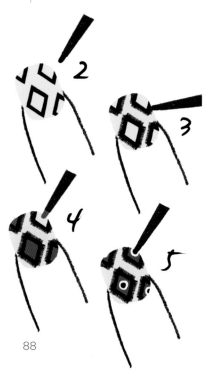

STEP 1 Manicure your nails with pale blue polish over a set basecoat and let it dry. While you're waiting, look at some ikat samples for inspiration—this fashion-forward fabric has been snagging fans for ages with its graphic shapes softened by blurred outlines, and there are tons of patterns and colors to choose from.

STEP 2 Lay out your aluminum foil palette and add a drop of black polish to it. Pick up some polish with your small, round paintbrush and paint diamond-shaped outlines for your ikat shapes on your nails. Don't worry about making these shapes perfect.

STEP 3 With quick, short strokes, paint tiny black lines over the edges of your diamonds on all your nails to give them that woven effect. Hot tip: Hold your paintbrush parallel to the nail for better results.

STEP 4 Gently dab pink polish in the center of each ikat shape using the bottle brush, filling the diamond with romantic, rosy color. Again, rough edges are best.

STEP 5 When this dries, rinse your round paintbrush and drop white polish in the pink spots' centers. After that's dry, too, add a drop of black polish to your palette, rinse your paintbrush again, and add a tiny dot inside each white spot.

STEP 6 Give your hippier-than-thou nails time to dry and slick on a clear topcoat. Let your free spirit roam.

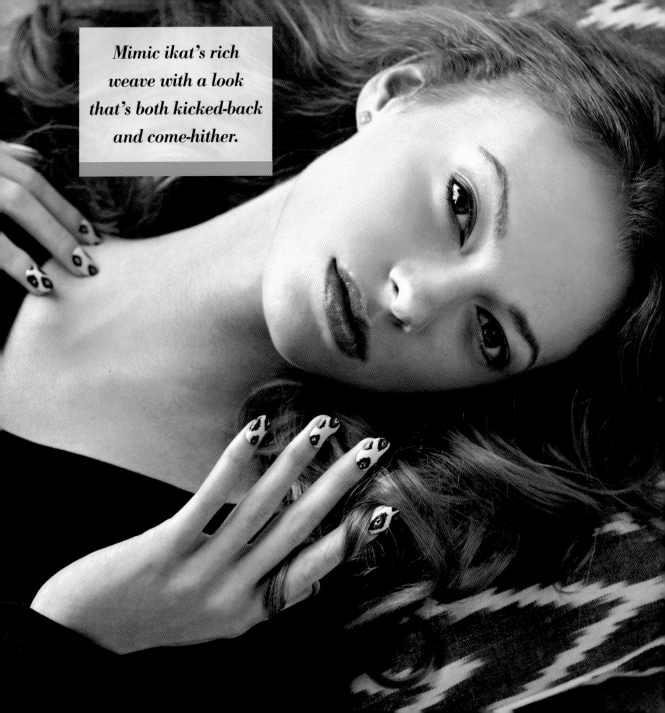

Mimic ikat's rich weave with a look that's both kicked-back and come-hither.

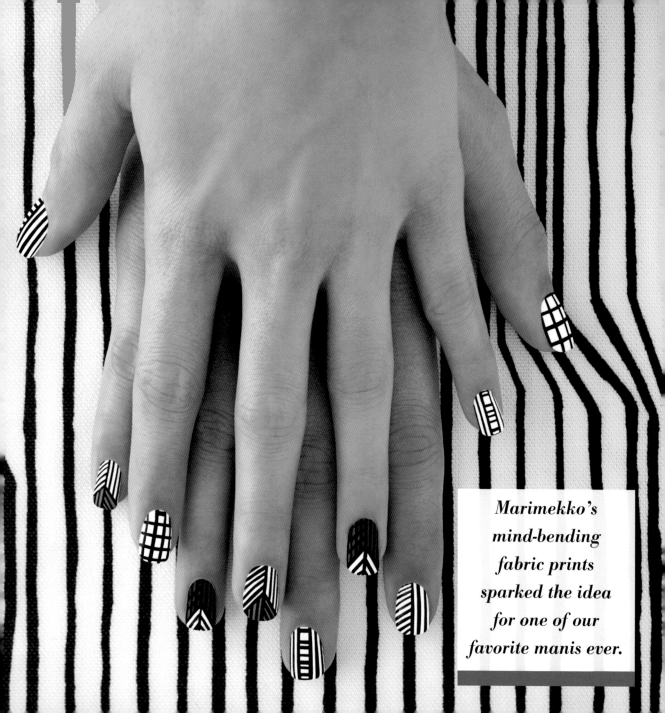

Marimekko's mind-bending fabric prints sparked the idea for one of our favorite manis ever.

PRINT ON A FUNKY Marimekko MANI

MATERIALS

BASECOAT

WHITE, RED, BLACK & BLUE POLISH

STRIPING BRUSH

CLEAR TOPCOAT

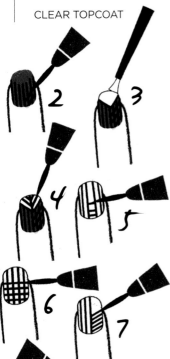

STEP 1 After you ABC (apply basecoat), paint all your nails except your ring fingers white. Paint those red and, while your 'tips dry, plot a pattern. This mani is all stripes, all the time. The trick is getting a mesmerizing mix on each hand!

STEP 2 Start with your red nails. Load your striping brush with black polish and paint vertical lines extending in a V shape two-thirds up the nail. When those are dry, cover one side of your nails with diagonal stripes. These stripes go from the nail's center to its sidewall, crossing your vertical stripes on their way.

STEP 3 Using the bottle brush, add white polish to the top of your red nail, then flare it out to make an inverted triangle at the tip. Repeat on your other red nail.

STEP 4 After these white triangles dry, lay down some black chevron stripes inside the white areas with your striping brush. Outline the white triangles, too.

STEP 5 Now it's time for your other nails! Pick two (we chose a pinky and middle finger), and paint four vertical lines on each with your striping brush. Two lines go on one side of the nail and the other two on the other side, leaving a gap in the middle. Fill this gap with horizontal stripes for a ladder effect.

STEP 6 Choose a couple of nails to put a grid on (we went with one index finger and one thumb). Grab your striping brush and lay down evenly spaced vertical stripes. When these dry, cross them with horizontal stripes.

STEP 7 Next, hit up your other index finger and thumb. Use that trusty striping brush to make one vertical stripe down the nails' centers. On one side of this line, paint vertical stripes. On the other side, go with diagonals.

STEP 8 Repeat the diagonal and vertical lines on your last two nails, stopping two-thirds up. Add blue polish near the tips and make inverted triangles, as you did on your red nails. Top off the blue with black vertical and diagonal stripes.

STEP 9 Let your nails dry, then finish off your handiwork with a clear topcoat.

SHAKE IT IN A Rock 'n' Roll LOOK

STEP 1 Over a dry basecoat, paint your pinkies and middle fingers white, index fingers blue, thumbs red, and ring fingers black.

STEP 2 While your nails dry, add silver and black polish to a piece of foil. Use a larger dotting tool to dot a silver Y shape down your black nail. Load a smaller dotting tool with black polish, then make two dots overlapping each dry silver dot for a zipper-tooth effect.

STEP 3 For the zipper pull, use a round paintbrush to paint a silver rectangle at the Y's intersection. Rinse your brush, dip it in black polish, and make a small square inside the rectangle near the Y intersection. Make a larger black rectangle under this square.

STEP 4 Use your striping brush to make a white cross on your blue nail. Then make a white X over the cross. Rinse your brush and paint narrow red stripes inside the white ones.

STEP 5 On your middle finger, swoop your small, round brush across the nail to outline the upper lip shape in red. From the corners of the mouth, draw the partial bottom lip and brazen stuck-out tongue. Fill in the tongue outline and let it all dry.

STEP 6 Rinse your small brush, dip it in black polish, and fill the mouth. Add a line to define the tongue and another one to separate the tongue from the bottom lip on the right side. When that's dry, rinse your brush and paint teeth and highlights on the tongue and top lip with white polish.

STEP 7 Paint your pinkies with glitter polish. For the killer glitter fade on your thumbs, stroke the glitter polish's brush back from the free edge toward the cuticle, concentrating glitter on the tip.

STEP 8 Let your look dry, add a topcoat, and give a record a spin.

92

MATERIALS

BASECOAT

WHITE, BLUE, RED, BLACK, SILVER & GLITTER POLISH

ALUMINUM FOIL

DOTTING TOOLS IN TWO SIZES

SMALL, ROUND PAINTBRUSH

STRIPING BRUSH

CLEAR TOPCOAT

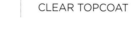
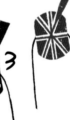
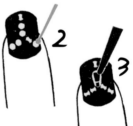
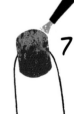
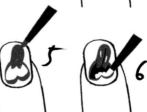

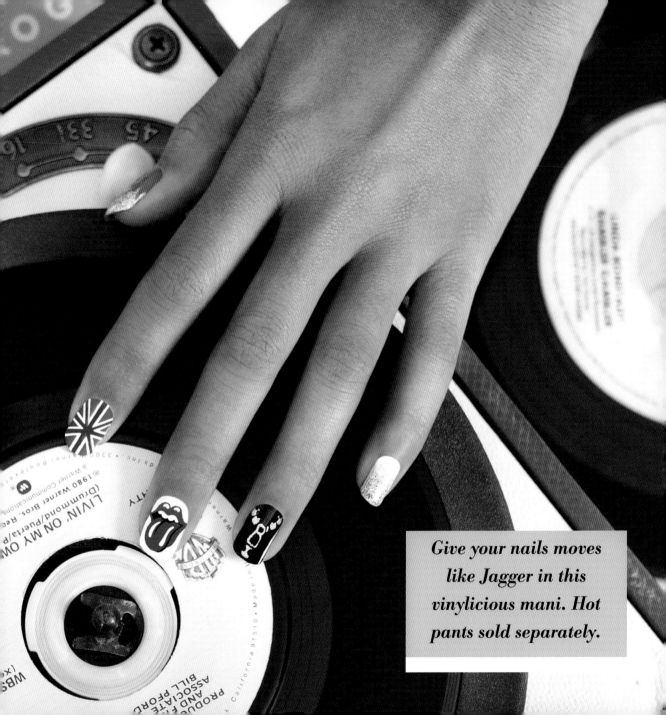

Give your nails moves like Jagger in this vinylicious mani. Hot pants sold separately.

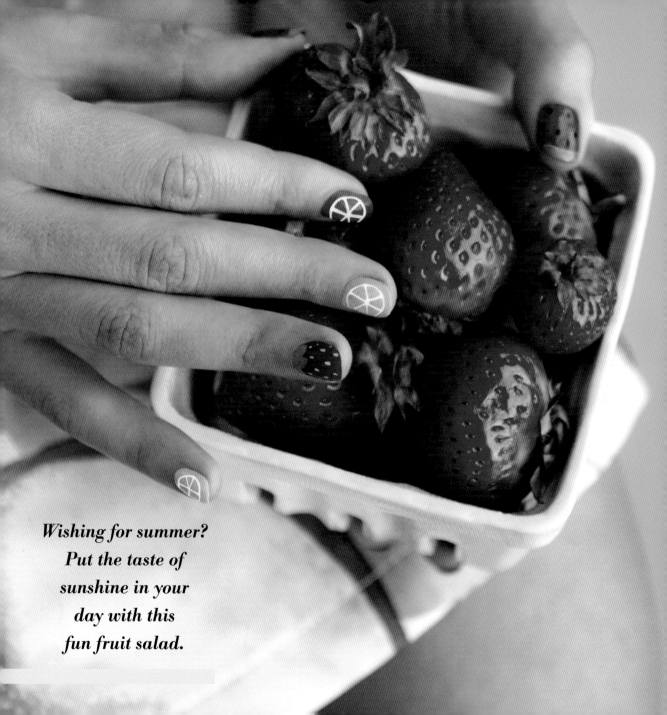

*Wishing for summer?
Put the taste of
sunshine in your
day with this
fun fruit salad.*

BITE INTO A Juicy Fruit MANI

STEP 1 Once your basecoat is dry, paint your thumbs deep pink, your index fingers orange, your middle fingers lime green, your ring fingers red, and your pinkies yellow. Let your nails dry.

STEP 2 Add leaf green polish to a piece of aluminum foil and pick up a small amount with your small, round paintbrush. Paint a zigzag outline around the cuticle areas of your ring fingers, filling in the outline for vibrant strawberry leaves.

STEP 3 Put a small drop of yellow nail polish on your foil palette. After rinsing your paintbrush, use its tip to make small yellow dots (you'll never have to pick these strawberry seeds out of your teeth!) all over your red nails.

STEP 4 Rinse your paintbrush and dip it into the leaf green polish on your palette. Paint a green swipe across the pink nails' tips to add a rind to your refreshing watermelon.

STEP 5 Add black polish to your palette. Rinse your brush and dip its tip in black polish, then use it to paint watermelon seeds over the pink base. Give your small paintbrush a rinse afterward.

STEP 6 Use an opaque white polish and its bottle brush to paint a white circle in the center of your orange, lime green, and yellow nails, filling in the circle. Let this dry.

STEP 7 Using the base color of each nail and your small paintbrush, make small triangles inside the white circles to create citrus segments. Let all your nails dry.

STEP 8 Finish off your fresh-from-the-farmers'-market mani with clear topcoat.

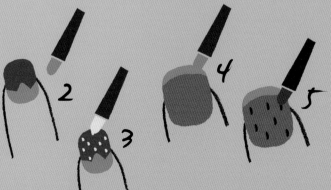

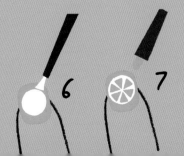

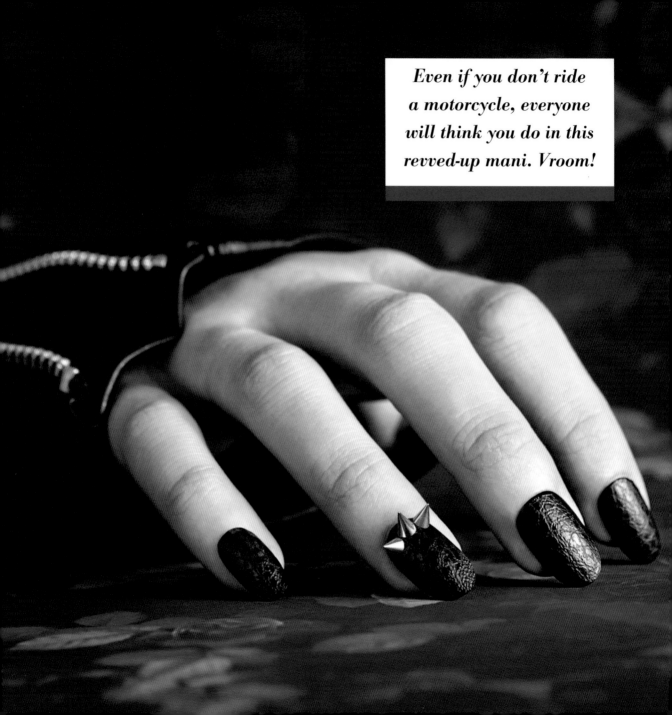

Even if you don't ride a motorcycle, everyone will think you do in this revved-up mani. Vroom!

STICK ON A TOUGH-GIRL
Leather Look

MATERIALS

SET OF FULL-COVERAGE
NAIL TIPS

ADHESIVE-BACKED LEATHER

PENCIL

SCISSORS

ORANGEWOOD STICK

EMERY BOARD

NAIL GLUE

TWEEZERS

6 SPIKES

STEP 1 Select fake nail tips that are about the size of your nails, filing them to fit if needed. (We like doing this look on a set of fake nails—this way, you don't get a lot of nasty adhesive on your natural nails.) Lay these onto the backside of your adhesive-backed leather and trace around them with a pencil.

STEP 2 Pick the nail tips up off the leather and then use scissors to cut out the leather nail shapes.

STEP 3 Peel back the protective backing from one of the leather shapes. Place it over its corresponding nail tip close to the bottom and adhere it, using the orangewood stick to press the leather smoothly onto the nail tip. Try a little nail glue if the leather lifts.

STEP 4 Trim the excess wrap hanging from the free edge with scissors and use an emery board to smooth out any rough edges. Hot tip: This press-on method works wonders with lots of adhesive textiles, like wood veneer, velvet, vinyl, or even wallpaper.

STEP 5 Use a drop of nail glue and tweezers to adhere your punk spikes wherever you choose. (We picked these up at a local piercing-supply store—you can hit up one near you for loads of edgy nail jewelry options.)

STEP 6 Affix your fake nails to your real ones with nail glue and continue your daily badassery.

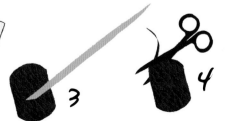

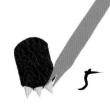

GO GRAPHIC IN A Comic Book MANI

STEP 1 Start with a dry basecoat, then paint your pinkies white, your ring fingers and thumbs red, one index finger yellow and the other blue, and one middle finger yellow and the other blue. Thumb through a comic or two while your nails dry.

STEP 2 Add yellow polish to a piece of foil. Use your small, round paintbrush to paint lightning bolts on your white nails.

STEP 3 Pour some white polish on the foil, rinse your brush, and paint speech bubbles on both blue nails and one red nail. Make some with squiggly edges, others with jagged shapes.

STEP 4 Turn your attention to your yellow nails. Rinse your paintbrush again and use it to paint white eyes on both nails, adding a small white oval at the corner of each eye for the tear. Fill the entire oval in with white polish. Let those eyes dry!

STEP 5 Now it's time for dots. Grab a dotting tool and sprinkle white dots on your blue nails, surrounding the speech bubbles. Rinse your tool and cover your other red nails with yellow spots.

STEP 6 Spill turquoise polish onto the foil, rinse your dotting tool, and make turquoise dots around the eyes on your yellow nails. Then add dots for the eye's iris. Let your nails dry.

STEP 7 Spill black polish onto your palette, rinse your brush, and dip it in black. Outline your speech bubbles, eyes, and lightning bolts, adding letters and exclamation points inside the bubbles and pupils and eyebrows to your eyes.

STEP 8 When your nails are completely dry, add a clear topcoat. Shazam! Our heroine wins the day.

MATERIALS

BASECOAT

WHITE, RED, YELLOW, BLUE, TURQUOISE & BLACK POLISH

ALUMINUM FOIL

SMALL, ROUND PAINTBRUSH

DOTTING TOOL

CLEAR TOPCOAT

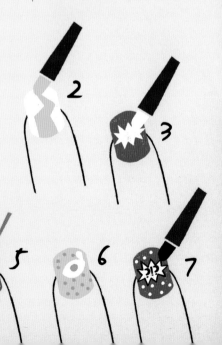

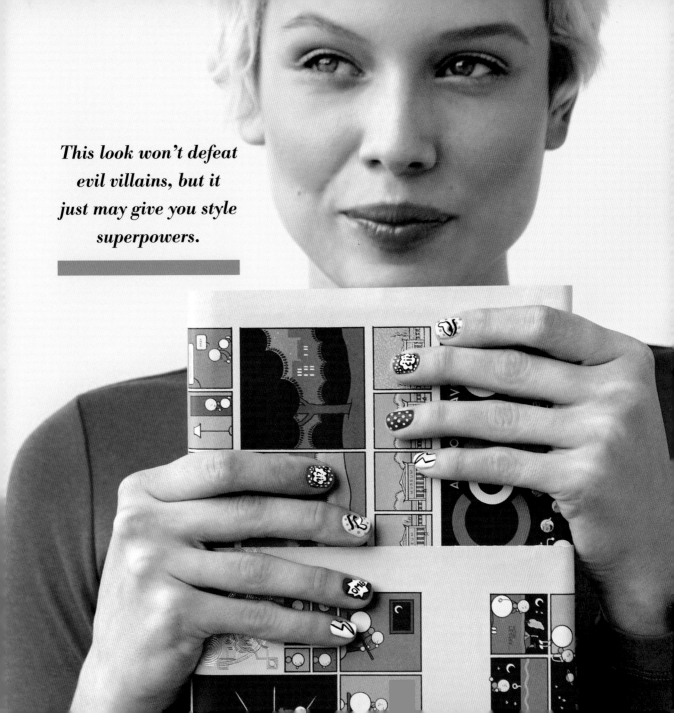

This look won't defeat evil villains, but it just may give you style superpowers.

SPAN THE GLOBE WITH Nomad NAILS

MATERIALS

- BASECOAT
- BEIGE & RED POLISH
- STRIPING BRUSH
- ALUMINUM FOIL
- SMALL, ROUND PAINTBRUSH
- CLEAR TOPCOAT

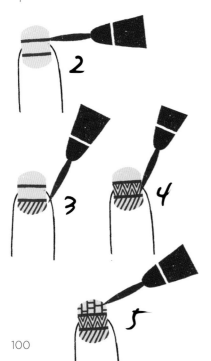

STEP 1 Start with your trusty basecoat, let it dry, and then paint on a quiet beige to create a subtle background for those loud stripes coming up.

STEP 2 Let your nails dry, and dip your striping brush into a bottle of red polish. Paint two horizontal stripes across your nails, dividing each nail into three parts. Hot tip: Creating zones makes your design simple to manage and cohesive to view.

STEP 3 Inside your first segment, use your striping brush to lay down some diagonal lines. Let this dry while you move on to do a section on each of your other nails, mixing up the pattern as you go.

STEP 4 Move on up to the second segment, trying a slightly different collection of lines or shapes, like these eye-catching zigzags. Hit your other nails up with fresh ideas in each section, too, and let them dry.

STEP 5 Paint the third section on all your nails with another variation on the theme, such as horizontal and vertical lines or even some curly swoops. (For more organic lines, spill polish onto a piece of foil and use a small, round paintbrush.) Try filling in a few shapes to play with negative space.

STEP 6 After your multilayered mani has dried, seal that radness in with a clear topcoat.

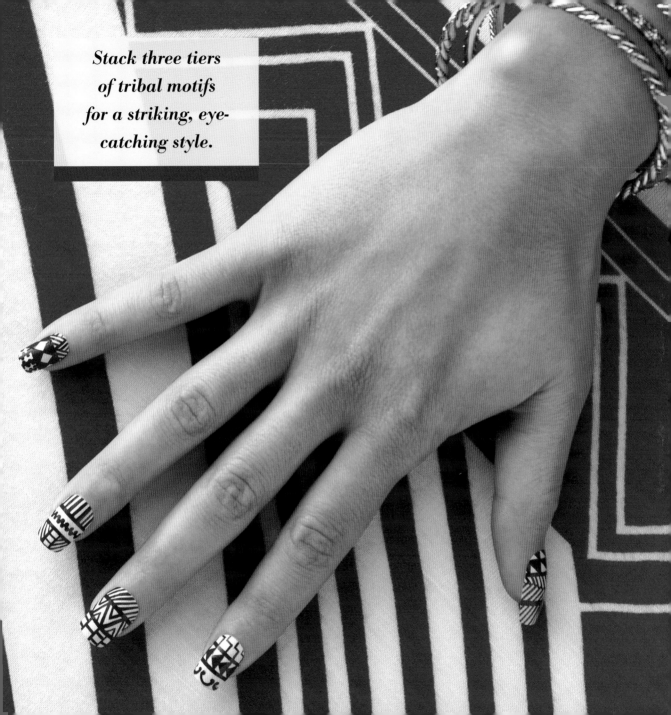

Stack three tiers of tribal motifs for a striking, eye-catching style.

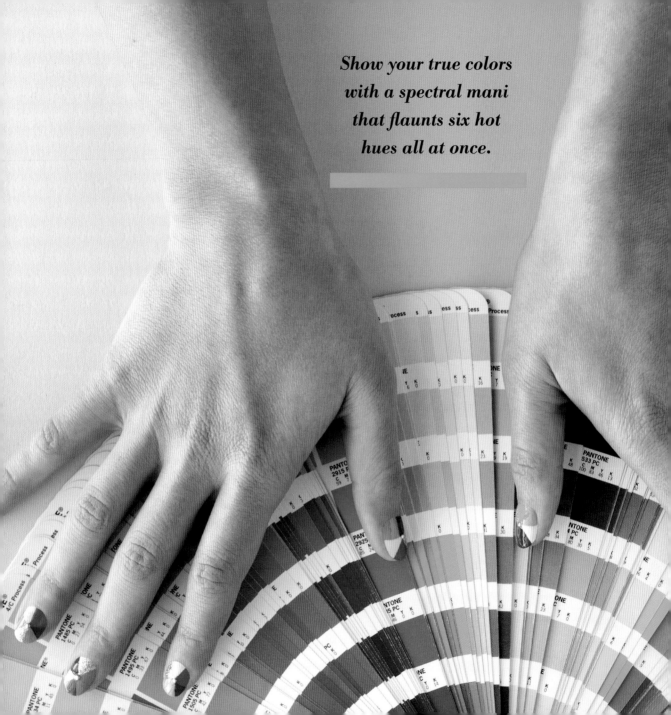

Show your true colors
with a spectral mani
that flaunts six hot
hues all at once.

ROLL OUT *Color Wheels*

MATERIALS

BASECOAT

ORANGE, YELLOW, RED, GOLD, GREEN & BLUE POLISH

ALUMINUM FOIL

SMALL, ROUND PAINTBRUSH

DOTTING TOOL

CLEAR TOPCOAT

10 GOLD STUDS

STEP 1 Do your ABCs (apply basecoat), then plan a color scheme while it dries: Try a few hues that are similar and some that contrast next to each other.

STEP 2 Pour some orange polish onto aluminum foil, then dip in your small, round paintbrush and place it in your first nail's center. Pull the brush out to the nail's edge to make one side of a triangle, then paint a second line to complete a triangle about one-sixth the size of your fingernail. Fill in this triangle with polish.

STEP 3 Make one triangle in this color on each fingernail, mixing up the color placement as you go.

STEP 4 Repeat with five more colors, covering all your nails with triangles and rinsing your brush between shades. Paint on a second coat of any color that's still translucent, then give your nails time to dry.

STEP 5 Use a dotting tool to place clear topcoat in the center of each nail where the color slices converge. Then, with the dotting tool, pick up gold studs one by one and press each into the topcoat, adding a pin to your pinwheel. Let your nails dry.

STEP 6 Slick on a layer of clear topcoat for a vibrant mani that's sure to make you dream in Technicolor.

THROW A *Picnic* FOR YOUR FINGERS

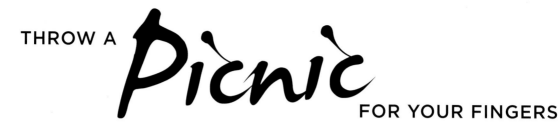

MATERIALS

BASECOAT

WHITE, BEIGE, RED, BLACK, BROWN, YELLOW & GREEN POLISH

ALUMINUM FOIL

SMALL, ROUND PAINTBRUSH

STRIPING BRUSH

DOTTING TOOLS IN THREE SIZES

CLEAR TOPCOAT

STEP 1 When your basecoat is dry, paint your pinkies, thumbs, and middle fingers white. Paint your hot dog and hamburger nails (ring and index) beige. Let those babies dry.

STEP 2 Add red polish to a piece of foil. Dip in your small, round paintbrush and paint small squares in a checkerboard pattern on your white nails. Next, paint thin, diagonal red stripes in the spaces between the red squares you just made, and let your nails dry.

STEP 3 Dribble black polish onto your foil. To make ants on your middle fingers, use three sizes of dotting tools to create a row of spots from largest to smallest.

STEP 4 Switch to your round paintbrush, give it a rinse, and paint six tiny black legs on each ant's body. Don't forget antennae!

STEP 5 Add yellow, green, brown, and more red polish to your foil for your hot dog and hamburger nails. Rinse your brush and make a brown squiggle down the middle of your hot dog nails. Let these dry, rinse again, and add squiggles of yellow and red, too.

STEP 6 Rinse, then make yellow, green, and red swipes across the center of your hamburger nails with your small, round paintbrush. When that's dry, use black polish and your striping brush to outline the layers of your burger, creating your bun.

STEP 7 Use your smallest dotting tool to add white dots in your hamburger nails' beige half-moon shape—sesame seeds!

STEP 8 Topcoat it up and fire up that grill.

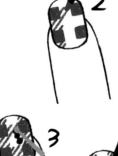

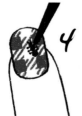

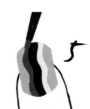

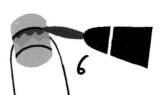

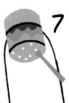

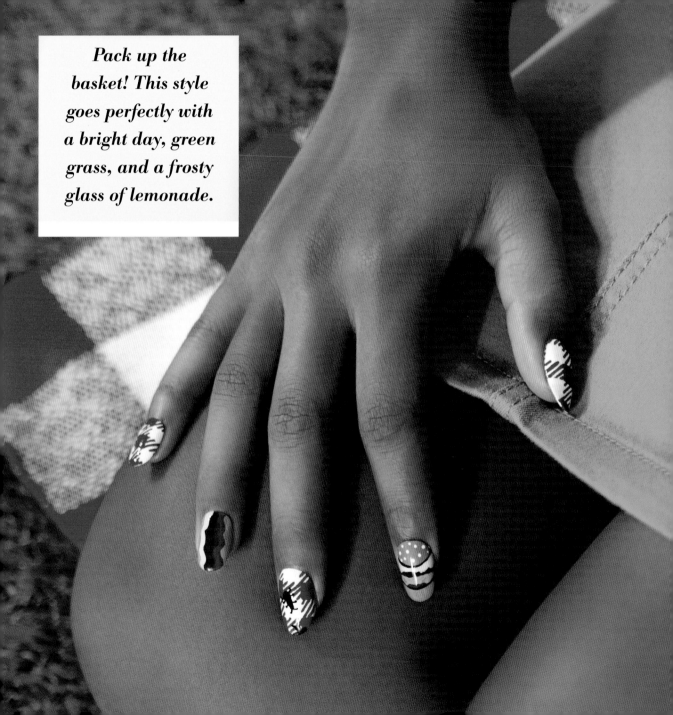

Pack up the basket! This style goes perfectly with a bright day, green grass, and a frosty glass of lemonade.

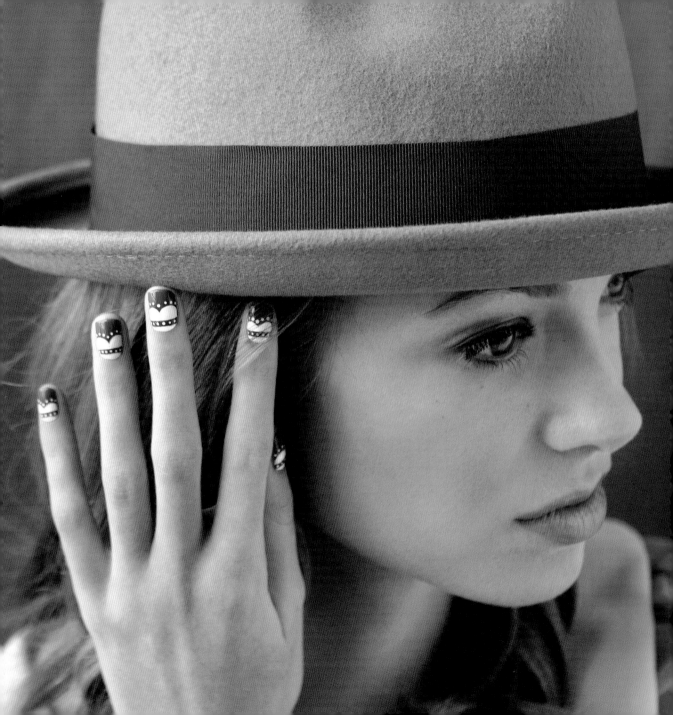

STROLL IN HIS SHOES WITH A *Wingtip* MANI

MATERIALS

BASECOAT

GREEN & WHITE POLISH

ALUMINUM FOIL

SMALL, ROUND PAINTBRUSH

STRIPING BRUSH

DOTTING TOOL

CLEAR TOPCOAT

STEP 1 After your basecoat has a chance to dry, lacquer your nails in a resonant green color.

STEP 2 Pour white polish onto a piece of foil. Dip your small, round paintbrush into the polish and nuzzle its tip into your nail's sidewall. Swoop the brush up and then down, making one half of a heart top. Repeat on the other side.

STEP 3 Fill in each nail below this half-heart shape with white. You may need an extra coat to keep that lush green polish from peeking through.

STEP 4 When your nails are dry, dip your striping brush in green polish and make a horizontal line across the base of each white half-heart shape.

STEP 5 Collect white polish on your dotting tool and outline the half-heart shape with circles to mimic wingtips' broguing. Place a row across the green horizontal stripe, too.

STEP 6 Once your wingtips are dry, slick on a layer of clear topcoat. Marlene Dietrich, eat your heart out.

Who knew your boyfriend's shoe rack was so chock-full of nail inspiration?

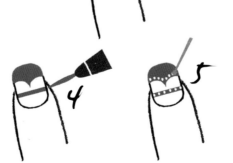

SETTLE INTO SUNDAYS WITH

Houndstooth

CHECKS

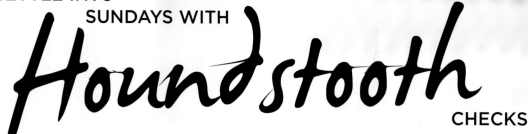

MATERIALS

BASECOAT

PALE BLUE & DARK BLUE POLISH

ALUMINUM FOIL

SMALL, ROUND PAINTBRUSH

CLEAR TOPCOAT

STEP 1 Don't forget your ABCs (apply basecoat). After it dries, paint your nails in your lighter color—we love the cozy coolness of light and dark blue, but pairing light and dark shades of any color will sing. The color secret to this mani is subtle contrast.

STEP 2 Let your nails dry, then pour some of your second color of nail polish onto your aluminum foil. Dip your round paintbrush in the polish and use it to paint a small square on your first nail.

STEP 3 Paint two teeny-tiny triangles barely overlapping one bottom corner of this square.

STEP 4 Use the tip of your brush to paint short, straight lines out from the two corners of the square adjacent to your triangles.

STEP 5 Add more houndstooth checks around the one you just made, continuing the pattern. Hot tip: Your checks should be spaced evenly on the nail so that they look like the real deal.

STEP 6 Repeat on all your nails and let them dry, then add clear topcoat, which'll slick over all those brushstrokes for a gleaming, smooth finish. Snuggle up with a cup of tea and a hard-boiled detective novel and you've got a recipe for the perfect Sunday afternoon.

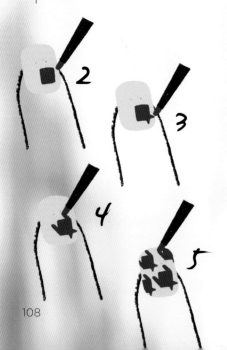

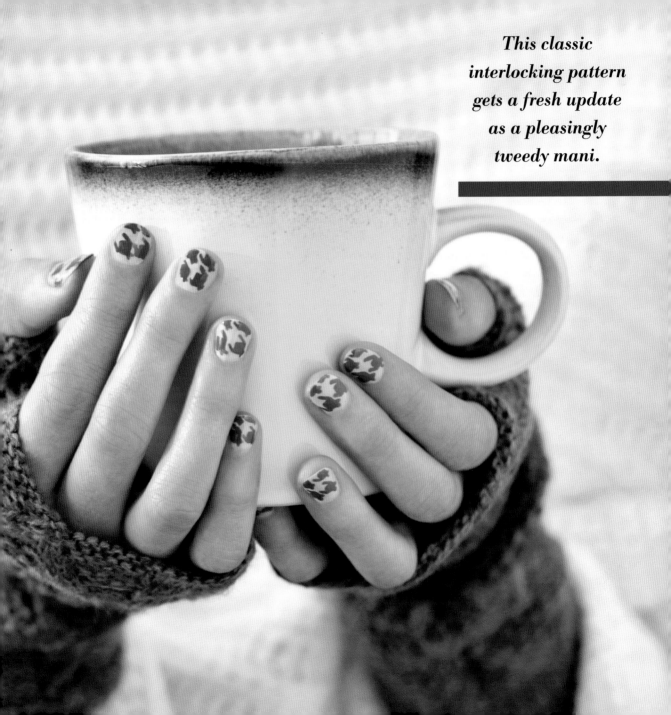

This classic interlocking pattern gets a fresh update as a pleasingly tweedy mani.

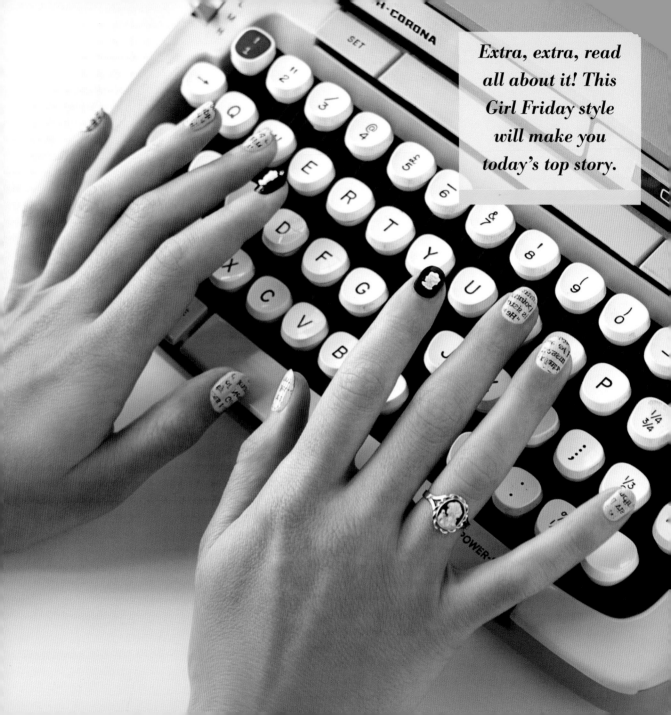

Extra, extra, read all about it! This Girl Friday style will make you today's top story.

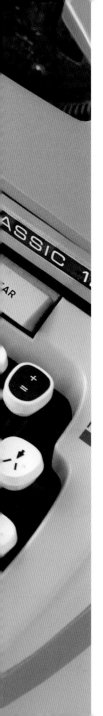

MAKE *Headlines* WITH YOUR MANI

MATERIALS

- NEWSPAPER OR ANY INK-PRINTED PAPER
- SCISSORS
- BASECOAT
- BLACK & PUTTY-COLORED POLISH
- WIDE, FLAT PAINTBRUSH
- DAPPEN DISH
- RUBBING ALCOHOL
- TWEEZERS
- CLEAR TOPCOAT
- 2 CAMEO EMBELLISHMENTS

STEP 1 Cut pieces of newspaper into bits that will cover your nails. Get creative—use magazines, printed designs, barcodes, photos of your celebrity crush, or old books for inspiration.

STEP 2 Over dry basecoat, paint your index fingers black and your other nails a putty color. (The light base color will give your nails that classic newsprint look, but these headlines will look great over colors like orange and yellow, too.) Once your look is dry, press a piece of newspaper onto a putty nail, ink side down.

STEP 3 Dip your wide, flat brush into your dappen dish of rubbing alcohol and brush it over your fingernail, being careful not to slide the piece of newspaper—that'll cause smudges. Don't stress if you smear a nail or two and have to re-do them; this ink-transfer process can be finicky.

STEP 4 Use the tweezers to gently peel off the paper, leaving behind the ink. Repeat this step on all your putty-colored nails and give them a chance to dry.

STEP 5 On your black nails, add topcoat in the center and use the tweezers to adhere a cameo to each for a feminine flourish.

STEP 6 Apply a layer of topcoat to all your nails to seal your ink.

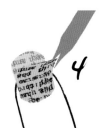

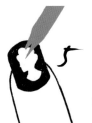

Go Incognito IN Camo

STEP 1 Start with a basecoat and let it dry, then paint on a beige or nude shade. Beige works best for these classic fatigue colors (which, trust us, are anything but tired), but you can also brighten it up with orange, pink, or light blue.

STEP 2 When your nails are dry, make a large puddle of army green polish on a piece of foil that will serve as your palette. Dip in the tip of your small, round paintbrush and paint the outlines of wobbly shapes on each nail.

STEP 3 Use the small, round paintbrush to fill in these shapes with the green polish. Rinse your brush when you're done.

STEP 4 Spill brown polish onto the palette and paint more wobbly shapes, bumping some against the green ones.

STEP 5 Add some black polish to your foil, rinse your brush again, and doodle shapes in some of the spaces between your green and brown shapes. Be sure to leave some of the nude areas uncovered for a true camo effect.

STEP 6 Lay on a matte topcoat for some unexpected sophistication. Drop and give us twenty!

MATERIALS

BASECOAT

BEIGE, ARMY GREEN, BROWN & BLACK POLISH

ALUMINUM FOIL

SMALL, ROUND PAINTBRUSH

MATTE TOPCOAT

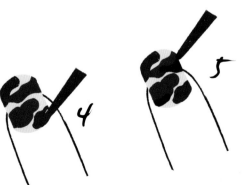

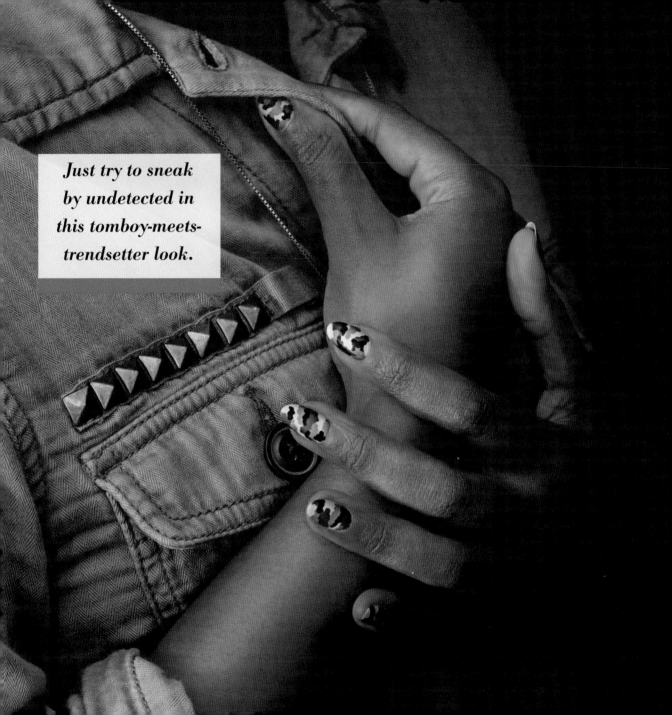

Just try to sneak by undetected in this tomboy-meets-trendsetter look.

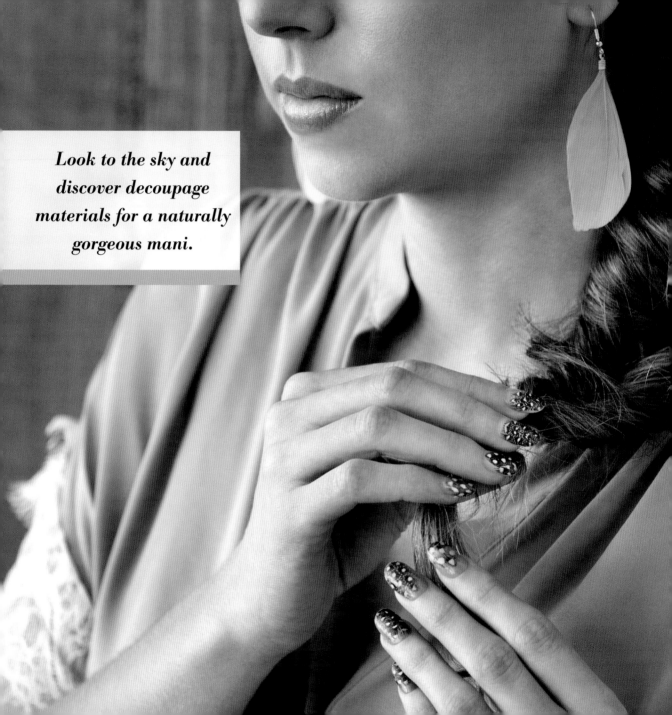

Look to the sky and discover decoupage materials for a naturally gorgeous mani.

LEARN TO FLY WITH

Feathery
FINGERTIPS

MATERIALS

MATERIALS

BASECOAT

NUDE POLISH

CLEAR TOPCOAT

PRETTY, PLIABLE
FEATHERS

SCISSORS

STEP 1 Do your ABCs (apply basecoat). When it's dry, add two coats of earthy-hued polish that's similar to your skin tone.

STEP 2 Apply one thin layer of clear topcoat and get started on your next step before it's completely dry, while it's still a little tacky.

STEP 3 Place a feather onto a nail with the feather tip (that'd be the soft, fluttery end) pointed toward the cuticle. Use your fingertip to press the feather onto the nail so it adheres evenly.

STEP 4 Gently tug at the quill end of the feather—this will help draw the feather fibers taut on your nail.

STEP 5 Use your scissors to trim off any excess plumage hanging over the edge of the nail. Repeat on each nail. Hot tip: This decoupage technique can be used with just about anything you want to glue onto your nails. Raid a craft store, which is where we scored these synthetic pheasant feathers—no birds were harmed in the making of this mani!

STEP 6 Apply another layer of topcoat to seal your look and smooth any stray fibers. Ca-caw!

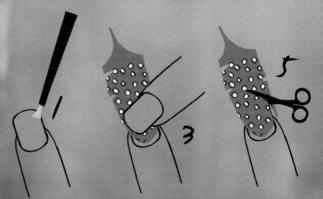

115

Shower Flowers

ALL OVER YOUR NAILS

MATERIALS

BASECOAT

BRIGHT PINK, WHITE, PURPLE & YELLOW POLISH

ALUMINUM FOIL

DOTTING TOOLS IN THREE SIZES

CLEAR TOPCOAT

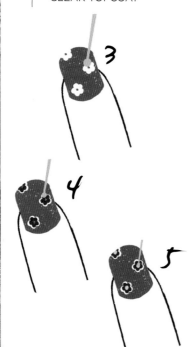

STEP 1 Start with a basic manicure in bright pink (over that dry basecoat you'd never forget to apply, of course).

STEP 2 Pour a small pool of white polish onto a piece of aluminum foil. Dip your largest dotting tool into this polish and, with even pressure, quickly place three dots in a half-circle on your first nail. The whole reason this mani is so much easier than it looks is that it's all dots—keep this technique in your pocket for other designs, too.

STEP 3 Dip your dotting tool into the white polish again and place two additional dots, completing a circle of five petals. Make as many petal circles as desired on all your nails. Let these dry.

STEP 4 Add purple polish to your foil palette, and dip in a smaller dotting tool. Make smaller purple dots inside all the white circles you just made. Let your purple petals dry.

STEP 5 Add some yellow polish to your palette. Dip in your smallest dotting tool and use it to make one tiny dot in the center of each flower.

STEP 6 Let your flowers dry, then add clear topcoat. You won't need a key to unlock this secret garden!

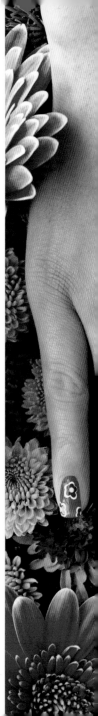

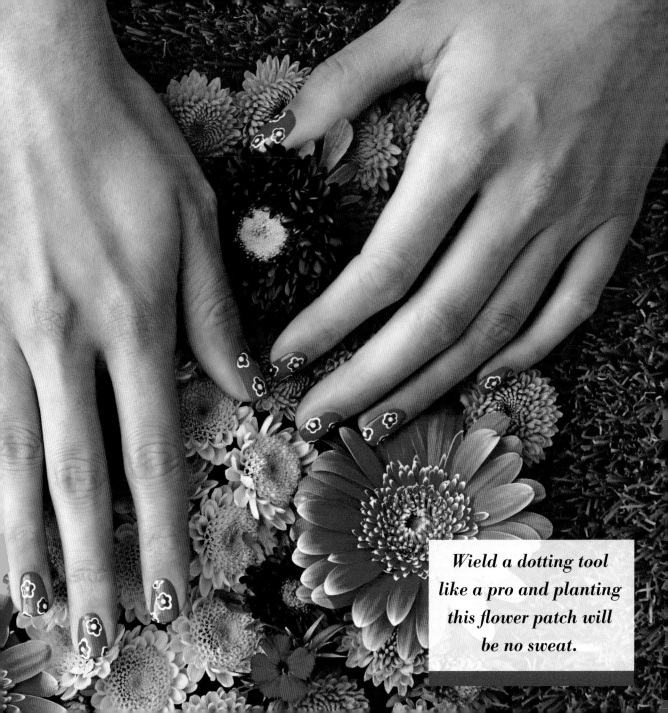

Wield a dotting tool like a pro and planting this flower patch will be no sweat.

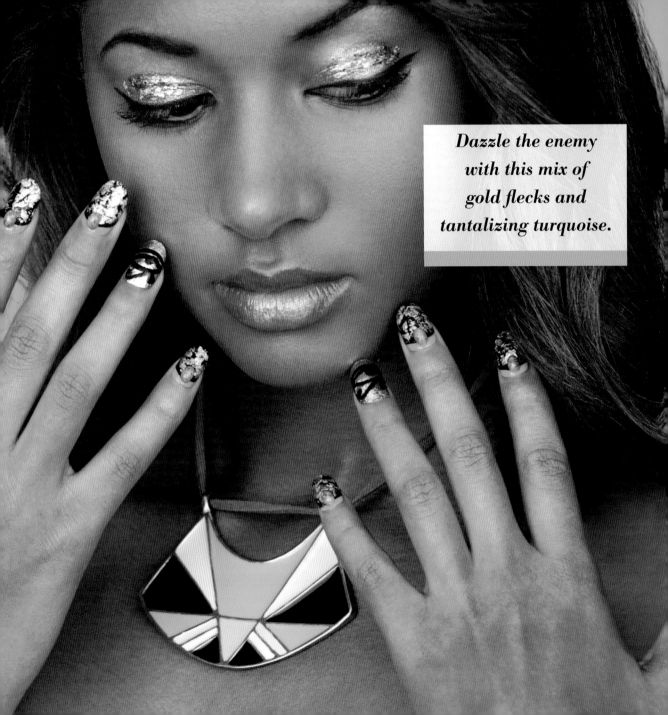

Dazzle the enemy with this mix of gold flecks and tantalizing turquoise.

Cleopatra

NAILS

MATERIALS

BASECOAT

GOLD, TURQUOISE
& BLACK POLISH

NAIL GLUE

WIDE, FLAT PAINTBRUSH

GOLD LEAF FLAKES

CLEAR TOPCOAT

DOTTING TOOL

8 FLAT-BACKED
TURQUOISE STONES

STRIPING BRUSH

ALUMINUM FOIL

SMALL, ROUND
PAINTBRUSH

STEP 1 Over a dry basecoat, paint your ring fingernails gold and the rest of your nails turquoise. Let them dry.

STEP 2 Open your black polish and press the brush's tip down near the cuticle of a turquoise nail. Sweep it toward one sidewall, then up to cover one half of the nail. Repeat on the other side and on your other turquoise nails for a cool reverse French.

STEP 3 Let your nails dry, then dab nail glue onto the black part of a nail. Use a wide, flat brush to pick up and brush on gold leaf pieces. Then repeat on your other turquoise-and-black nails.

STEP 4 Use a dotting tool to dab clear topcoat in the blue area's center, then pick up a flat-backed turquoise stone and stick it to the nail. Add stones to your other turquoise-and-black nails, too.

STEP 5 Find flakes of gold leaf large enough to cover your ring finger accent nails. Brush each gold nail with nail glue—just keep it off your skin!—then apply the gold leaf pieces to the nail. Let it set, then flake off excess around the edges with your wide brush.

STEP 6 To paint the eye of Horus, dip your striping brush into black polish. Sweep the brush between the sidewalls to create two long, curved top and bottom lids. Add a third line for a dramatic brow and repeat the process on your other accent nail.

STEP 7 Pour black polish onto a piece of foil. On each accent nail, paint a curved swoop under the eye with a small, round paintbrush, then draw a triangle down from where the swoop begins. Fill it with polish and make a dot for the eye's iris.

STEP 8 Let your nails dry. Protect your riches with clear topcoat.

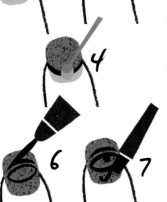

119

PEEK INTO A
Stained Glass

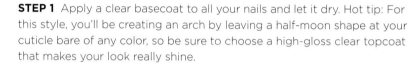

MANI

MATERIALS

CLEAR BASECOAT

RED, YELLOW, ORANGE, PINK, BLUE, TEAL & PURPLE JELLY POLISH

ALUMINUM FOIL

DOTTING TOOL

DENSE GLITTER POLISH

SMALL, ROUND PAINTBRUSH

CLEAR TOPCOAT

STEP 1 Apply a clear basecoat to all your nails and let it dry. Hot tip: For this style, you'll be creating an arch by leaving a half-moon shape at your cuticle bare of any color, so be sure to choose a high-gloss clear topcoat that makes your look really shine.

STEP 2 Place a few random dots of your first jelly polish on each fingernail—this polish dries slightly translucent, making it perfect for our stained glass effect. Use the bottle brush for larger dots, or add polish to a piece of foil and use a dotting tool to make smaller, regular shapes.

STEP 3 Dot on as many more colors as you like, alternating large expanses of hue with tinier flecks and making sure to leave a bit of space between each segment. Don't even dream of filling in those bare arches on your nails' moons! Let your nails dry.

STEP 4 Place a dab of glitter polish on the foil. Pick some glitter polish up with your small, round paintbrush and trace around each spot of color.

STEP 5 Give your nails some time to dry, then slick on a clear topcoat for a mani made in heaven.

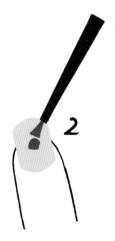

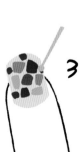

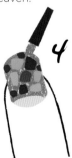

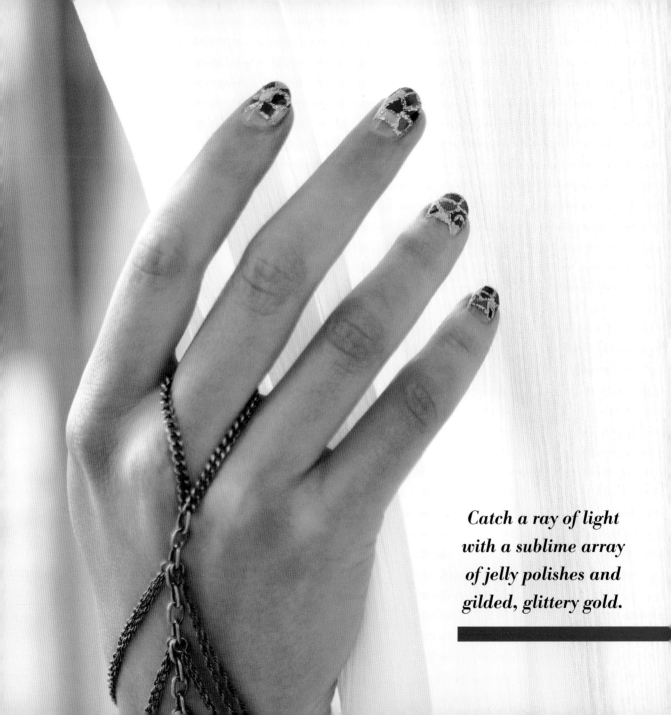

*Catch a ray of light
with a sublime array
of jelly polishes and
gilded, glittery gold.*

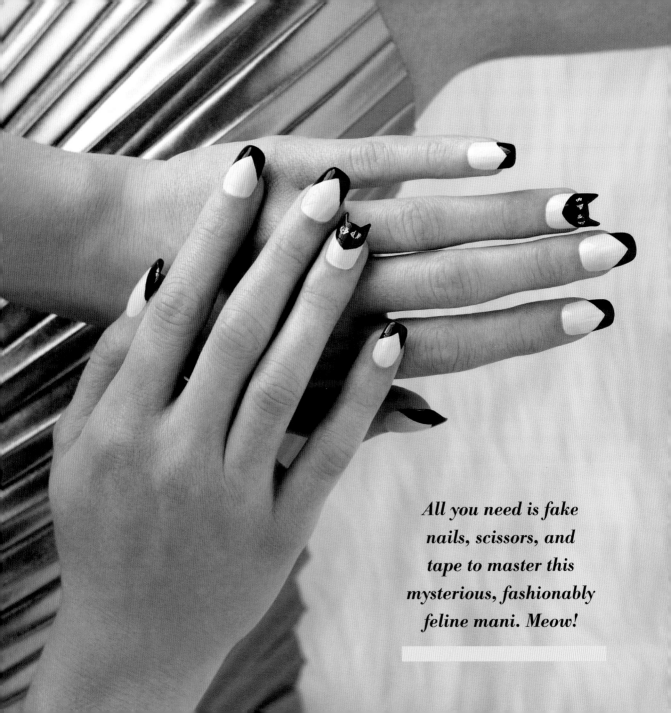

All you need is fake nails, scissors, and tape to master this mysterious, fashionably feline mani. Meow!

UNLEASH YOUR INNER Glamourpuss

MATERIALS

SET OF FULL-COVERAGE NAIL TIPS

PENCIL

SMALL SCISSORS

EMERY BOARD

BASECOAT

PALE PINK, BLACK & SILVER POLISH

TAPE

ALUMINUM FOIL

SMALL, ROUND PAINTBRUSH

CLEAR TOPCOAT

NAIL GLUE

STEP 1 Size your nail tips so that they fit snugly on each of your fingernails. For the kitty-face accent nails (we chose both ring fingers), mark the edge of your real nails onto the fake nails' backs with a pencil. Crucial hot tip: Do not attempt this mani on real nails.

STEP 2 To cut your kitty-face fake nails into the shape of cat ears, use small scissors to slice down at an angle on either side of each nail, cutting to the mark that you made on the fake nails' backs.

STEP 3 To make it easy to remove the center section between your cat ears, cut straight down inside your angled lines, meeting them at the mark you made to cut out two little triangles.

STEP 4 Finally, cut straight between the triangles to detach the center section. Use your emery board to smooth out all edges—no scratching!

STEP 5 Over a dry basecoat, paint your fake nails pale pink and let them dry. Cut twenty pieces of tape and arrange two in a deep, downward-facing V on your kitty-face fake nails. Position the other tape pieces into upward-facing Vs on the other fake nails, masking off angled French tips.

STEP 6 Paint the tops of the tips black; let them dry. Pull off the tape.

STEP 7 Pour silver polish onto a foil palette. With your small, round paintbrush, make one cat eye, painting two triangles on the left side of the face with a gap in between them. Repeat on the face's right side for a full set of peepers, then make eyes on the other kitty-face nail. Let dry.

STEP 8 Topcoat it up for super shine and attach your fake nails to your natural nails with nail glue. You're now the most elegant cat lady ever.

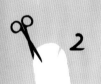 2

 3

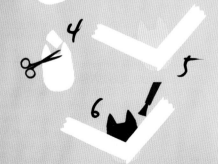 4 5

6

 7

LIFT THAT PINKY,

China Girl

STEP 1 Apply your traditional basecoat (trust us, this is one look that's all about tradition!) and let it dry. Then cover your nails in a white or creamy porcelain glaze and let them dry.

STEP 2 Pour a dot of cobalt blue polish onto your foil palette, then start a flower by dipping your dotting tool in blue and placing one dot on your first nail. Then create a circle of petals around the first dot. Repeat this process as many times as you like, creating fancy flowers of various sizes on all your nails.

STEP 3 Add vines and stems by using your small, round paintbrush to connect your flowers with sweeping, curved lines of cobalt polish.

STEP 4 Dip a striping brush into the polish and add leaves to the vines with light, short strokes.

STEP 5 Let your design dry and brush on a layer of clear topcoat. Don't forget to pass the crumpets, Princess.

MATERIALS

BASECOAT

WHITE & COBALT POLISH

ALUMINUM FOIL

DOTTING TOOL

SMALL, ROUND PAINTBRUSH

STRIPING BRUSH

CLEAR TOPCOAT

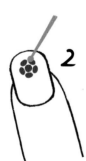
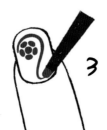
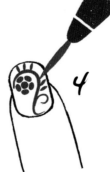

Hit high tea with a prim-and-proper pattern that's fit for the royals.

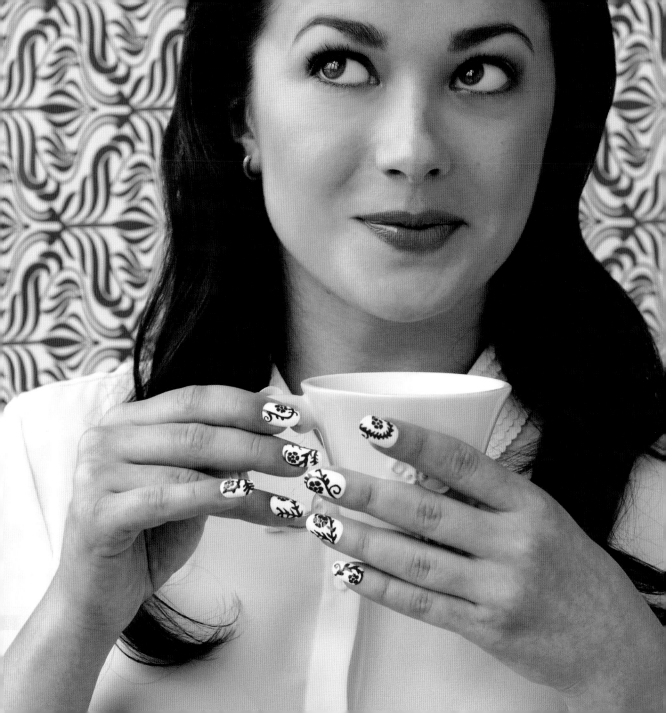

COVER YOUR 'TIPS WITH 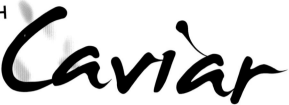 Caviar

MATERIALS

BASECOAT

MINT GREEN POLISH

CLEAR TOPCOAT

SMALL DISH FOR DIPPING

MINT GREEN CAVIAR
MICROBEADS

STEP 1 Begin with your ABCs (apply basecoat). After it dries, layer on a basic manicure in a shade of your choice—we fell hard for this fresh mint. Let it dry.

STEP 2 Paint clear topcoat over a fingernail that you want to cover with caviar. Here we've kept it simple by using the fancy stuff on only two accent nails, but you can make this look as luxe as you want, of course! Be ready to work with the topcoat while it's still tacky.

STEP 3 Fill a small dish with mint-colored micro-beads, then drop your finger, nail side down, into it.

STEP 4 Remove your finger from the dish and use the pad of a finger to gently push the beads around for full coverage, pressing them into the topcoat.

STEP 5 Apply a final layer of fast-drying topcoat on your other nails to seal in the drama. No need to hunt down the party—with this look, the party follows you.

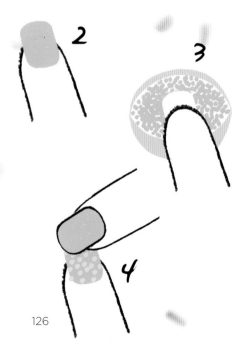

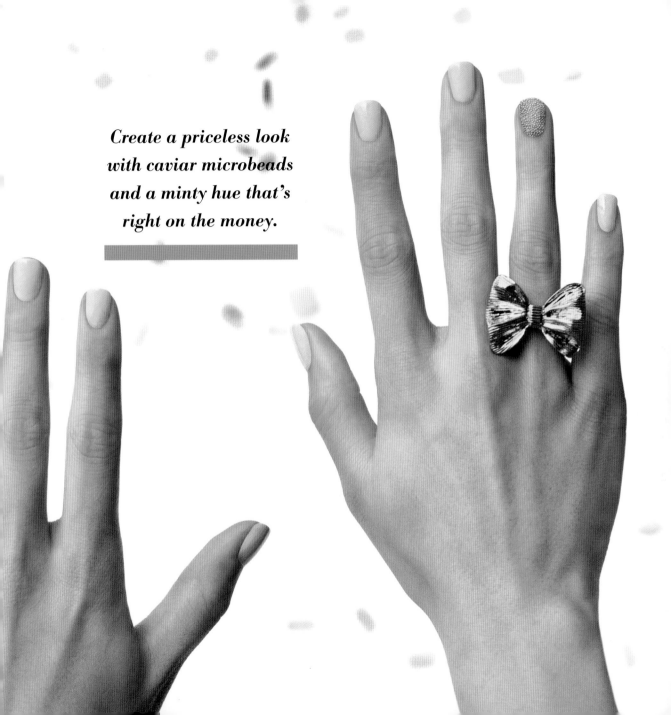

Create a priceless look with caviar microbeads and a minty hue that's right on the money.

DRIP ON A DREAMY

Watercolor Mani`

MATERIALS

BASECOAT

WHITE, YELLOW, RED
& BLUE POLISH

WIDE, FLAT PAINTBRUSH

DAPPEN DISH

ACETONE

CLEAR TOPCOAT

Très Monet! This beautifully blended mani covers nails in an impressionistic wash of colors.

STEP 1 Start with a basic mani in a light, opaque shade (we used pure white) over your dry basecoat. Let that dry.

STEP 2 Open up your polishes and use the bottle brushes to drop multicolored dots on your first nail. There's no need to make these dots too precise, as you're about to run them all together into a mini-masterpiece.

STEP 3 While your dots are still wet, dip your wide paintbrush into the dish of acetone. Lightly brush acetone onto the nail, smearing, spreading, diluting, and blending the colored dots.

STEP 4 Repeat on all of your nails, mixing up the color placement and dot size for an assortment of looks.

STEP 5 Watercolor the rest of your nails, let them dry, and protect your art with a clear topcoat.

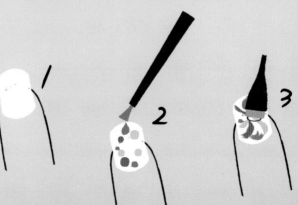

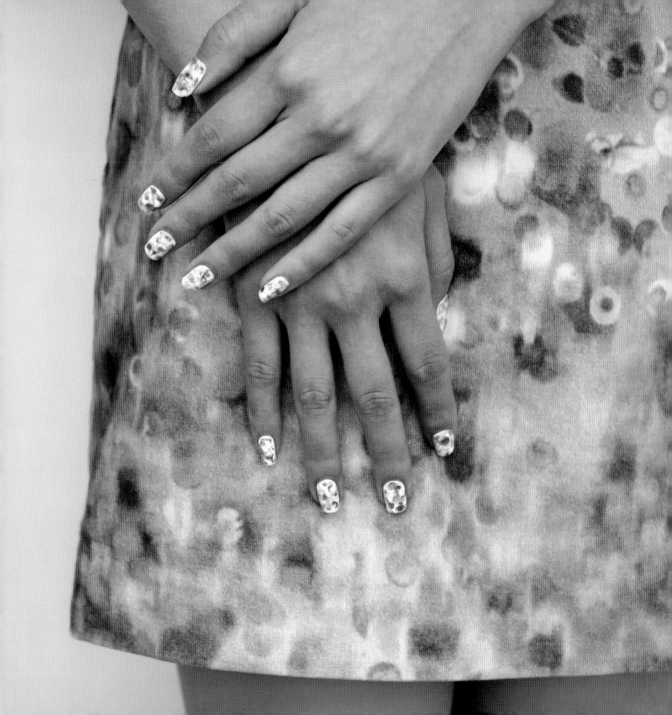

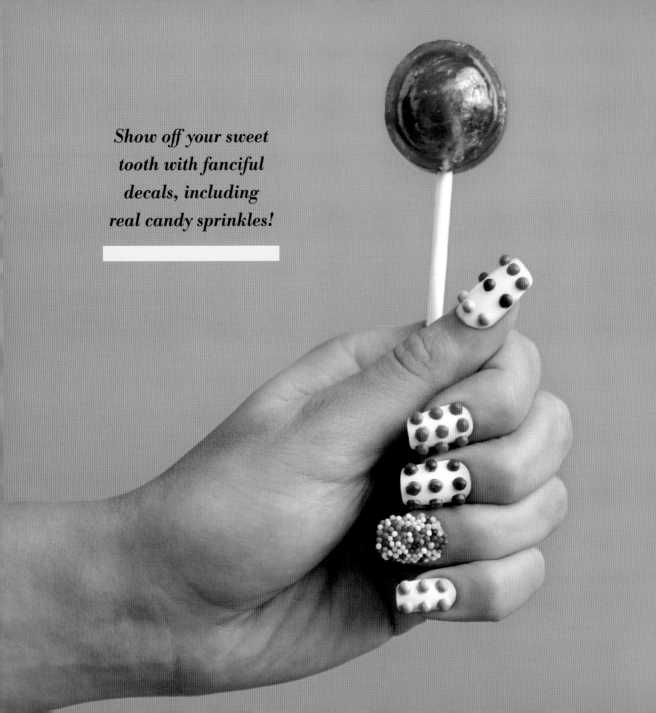

Show off your sweet tooth with fanciful decals, including real candy sprinkles!

SOAR ON A Sugar High WITH CANDYCOATED 'TIPS

STEP 1 Begin by wrapping a strip of tape around a buffing block or other cube-shaped item so that the sticky side faces out. Place rows of pearls total onto the tape so they'll stay in place while you paint them.

STEP 2 Paint 24 of the flat-backed pearls pink, 24 blue, and 18 yellow. Once they're dry, peel them off the tape and make sure each edge is clean.

STEP 3 Over a dry layer of basecoat, paint all your fingernails white and let them dry completely.

STEP 4 Brush clear topcoat onto a middle fingernail and use your dotting tool (with a dab of topcoat on its tip) to pick up one blue pearl. Place it onto the topcoat and press down firmly to seal it to your nail. Repeat to create rows of pearl candy dots, then repeat on your other middle finger.

STEP 5 Use the same process on your pinky fingers with yellow pearls. Place the pink pearls on your index fingers. On your thumbnails, mix up the colors into candy stripes.

MATERIALS

TAPE

BUFFING BLOCK

66 FLAT-BACKED PEARLS

PINK, BLUE, YELLOW & WHITE POLISH

BASECOAT

CLEAR TOPCOAT

DOTTING TOOL

ROUND RAINBOW CANDY SPRINKLES

SMALL DISH FOR DIPPING

STEP 6 Pour your candy sprinkles into a small container. Brush a layer of topcoat over your ring fingernails and dip them into the candy sprinkles.

STEP 7 Gently press the sprinkles into the topcoat. No nibbling allowed!

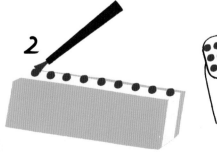
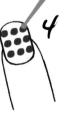
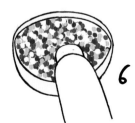
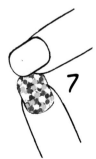

TRICK THE EYE IN *Turquoise*

MATERIALS

BASECOAT

DARK BROWN, LIGHT TURQUOISE, DARKER TURQUOISE & METALLIC GOLD POLISH

SMALL, ROUND PAINTBRUSH

SMALL BALL OF CRUMPLED CLING WRAP

CLEAR TOPCOAT

STEP 1 Paint all of your nails to perfection with dark brown polish over a dry basecoat.

STEP 2 Once your base color has dried completely, crumple a small piece of cling wrap into a ball. Paint splotches of each turquoise shade on one side of the crumpled ball.

STEP 3 Blot this side of the ball against your first fingernail to distribute the polish unevenly. Repeat on all nails until splotched with turquoise, adding more polish to the cling wrap as needed. Let this dry. Hot tip: Repeat if you're after more vibrant results.

STEP 4 To mimic a delicate ring setting, dip your small, round paintbrush into metallic gold polish and outline all the way around the perimeter of each fingernail.

STEP 5 When your gold polish has dried, brush on a layer of clear topcoat to perfect your nails' mineral sheen.

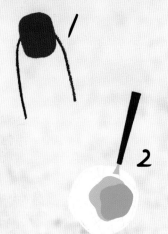

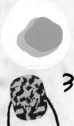

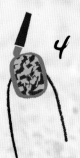

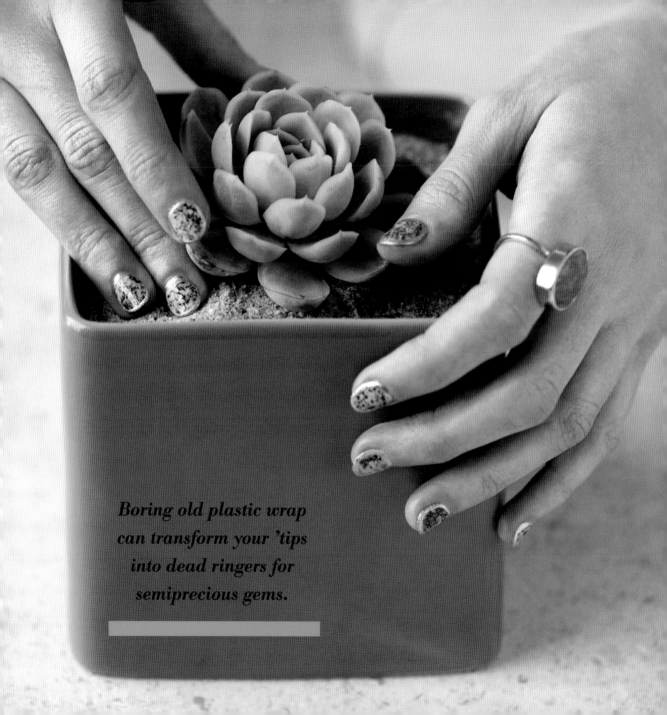

Boring old plastic wrap can transform your 'tips into dead ringers for semiprecious gems.

Extraterrestrial

'TIPS

STEP 1 Mind your ABCs, then cover your nails with a deep matte green shade that boasts a subtle intergalactic sheen. Let your nails dry.

STEP 2 Brush another coat of green polish onto the first nail. Use your dotting tool (with green polish on its tip) to stick a pearl onto the nail, then grab another pearl and repeat until you've made a row of five in the nail's center.

STEP 3 Paint your green polish over the pearls, then repeat the pearling and painting process on your other nails.

STEP 4 When your nails are dry, add a final layer of green polish to cover up any gaps between the pearls' edges and the nails' surface. This last layer is all you need—just this once, skip the clear topcoat and get beamed straight up.

MATERIALS

BASECOAT

MATTE, SHIMMERY
DARK GREEN POLISH

DOTTING TOOL

50 FLAT-BACKED PEARLS

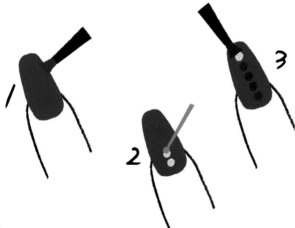

Land a futuristic alien look with some head-turning texture and an otherworldly flat shimmer.

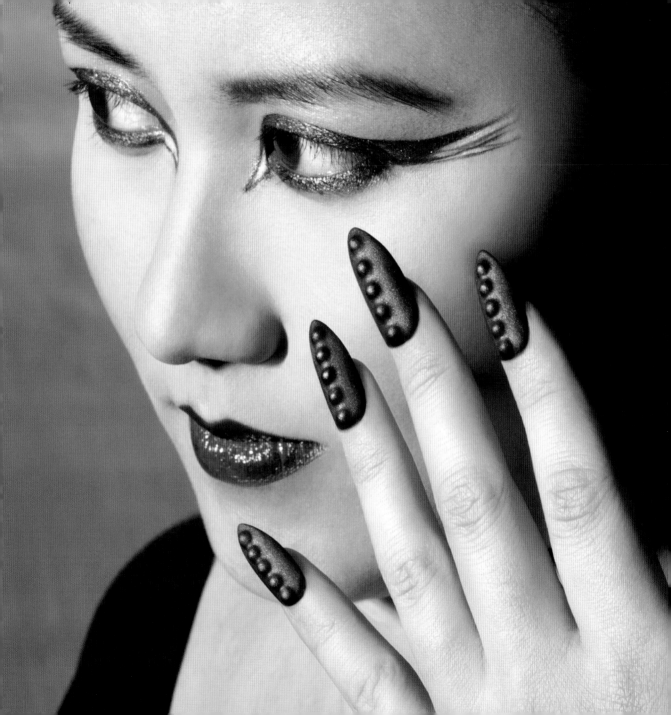

Index

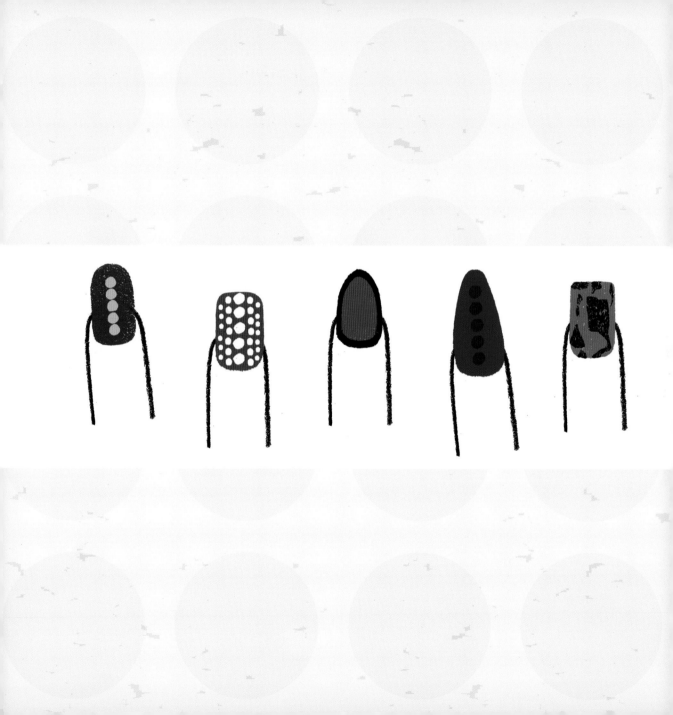

INDEX

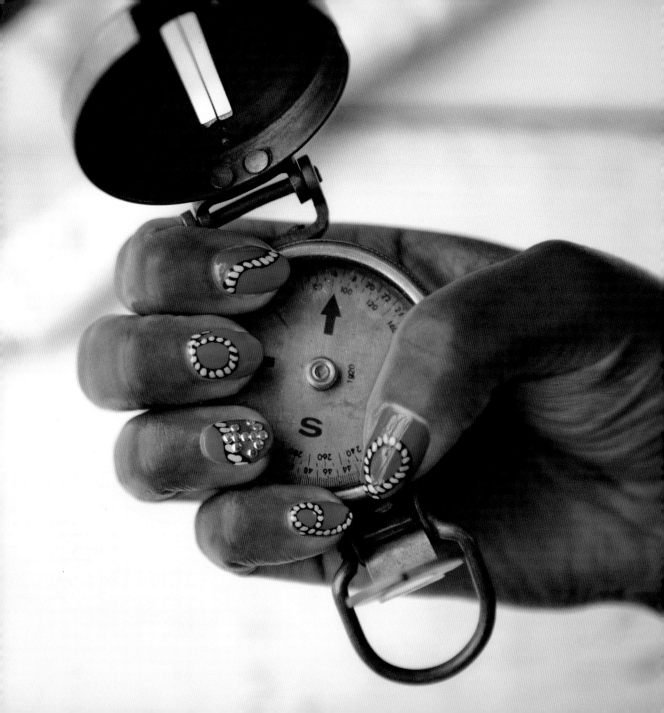

weldon**owen**

President, CEO **Terry Newell**
VP, Sales **Amy Kaneko**
VP, Publisher **Roger Shaw**
Senior Editor **Lucie Parker**
Project Editor **Emelie Griffin**
Contributing Editor **Laura Goode**
Creative Director **Kelly Booth**
Art Director **Lisa Milestone**
Designer **Michel Gadwa**
Illustration Specialist **Conor Buckley**
Production Director **Chris Hemesath**
Production Manager **Michelle Duggan**

415 Jackson Street, Suite 200
San Francisco, CA 94111

Telephone: 415 291 0100
Fax: 415 291 8841
www.weldonowen.com

Weldon Owen is a division of **BONNIER**

Copyright © 2013 Weldon Owen Inc.

All rights reserved, including the right of reproduction in whole or in part in any form

Library of Congress Control Number is on file with the publisher.

ISBN 13: 978-1-61628-492-3
ISBN 10: 1-61628-492-7

10 9 8 7 6 5 4 3 2 1
2013 2014 2015 2016 2017

Printed in China by 1010 Printing.

Photographs by Nicole Hill Gerulat, prop styling by Mallory Ullman, and illustrations by Debbie Powell.

Page 93: Rolling Stones Tongue and Lip Logo® Musidor B.V. Printed with permission.

ACKNOWLEDGMENTS

Weldon Owen would like to thank Laura Harger, Marianna Monaco, Katharine Moore, Katie Schlossberg, and Marisa Solís for editorial assistance, and Celeste Giuffre, Megan Peterson, Jenna Rosenthal, and Stephanie Tang for design help. We'd also like to thank photo assistant Lauren Andersen, stylist assistant Meredith Robinson, and hair and makeup artist Amy Lawson and her assistant Jennifer Pons for gorgeous looks.

Finally, we would like to give special thanks to our models and modeling agencies: Bria Adams, Exalt Model and Talent, Bridget Fitzgerald, Emelie Griffin, Lauren Inderkum, Gavyn Jones, Rhiannon Jordan, Naseem Khalili, Models Inc. Talent Agency, Amanda Nour, Lucie Parker, Alyssa Phan, Emma Rogers, Katie Schlossberg, Ellie Shaw, Candace Sims, and Mary Zhang.

ABOUT THE AUTHORS

Sisters Donne and Ginny Geer have turned their passion for nail art into a way of life. Their nail salon in Long Beach, California—Hey, Nice Nails!—serves as a haven for anyone seeking more than the average manicure, and fans outside of California can get their fix browsing the sisters' blog tutorials or their daily Instagram shots. The young entrepreneurs and licensed beauticians have been featured in such publications as The Huffington Post, *Allure, Marie Claire,* StyleList, and MTV's Style blog, and they've been raved about throughout the happening nail-art blogosphere. From elegant to funky to downright silly, the duo's nail designs are like candy to a generation of girls.

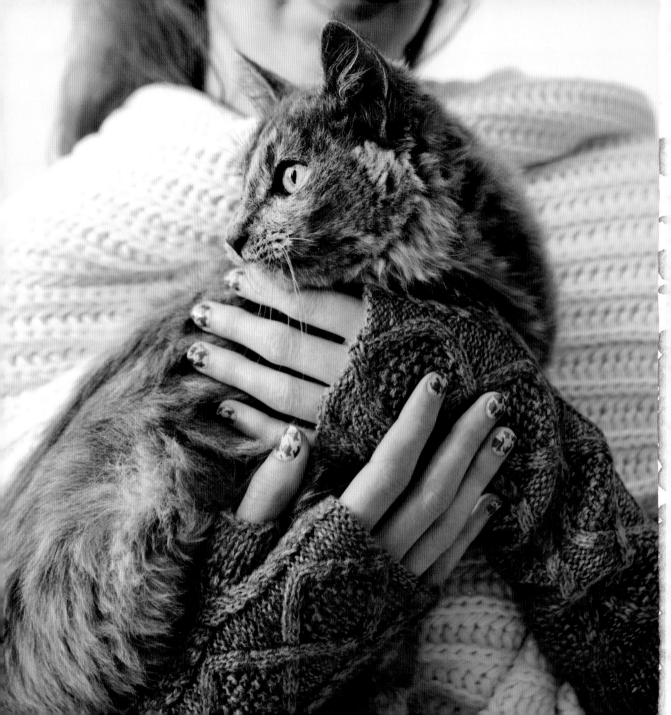